Living together as partners

THE ALTERNATIVE MARRIAGE GUIDE

MATTHEW JANES

foulsham

LONDON • NEW YORK • TORONTO • SYDNEY

foulsham

The Publishing House, Bennetts Close, Cippenham,
Berkshire, SL1 5AP, England

ISBN 0-572-02764-8

Printed in Great Britain by St. Edmundsbury Press, Bury St. Edmunds, Suffolk.

contents

introduction

This book is a straightforward and down-to-earth guide for couples who intend to spend their lives together but who are not married and do not intend to get married. For a variety of reasons, living together outside marriage is on the increase. Whether we approve or not, as a society – or as individuals – cohabiting is here to stay and is the preferred lifestyle choice for many couples.

The aim of this book is to offer practical advice not only to those couples contemplating sharing their lives in this way but also to those who already enjoy an intimate and fulfilling relationship under the same roof.

Some people think that living together is an easy and convenient option – rather like marriage but without all the strings attached. Wrong. Like all relationships, living together has its own unique set of problems and pressures that must be worked at by both partners to make it successful. If you are prepared to do this, however, there is no reason why you should not have an enduring and satisfying future together.

Your prime motive for living with someone is – or should be – driven by love and the desire to be with that special person constantly. However, as in a formal marriage, the ups and downs of everyday life can soon intrude on even the most harmonious of relationships. In writing this book, I have tried to offer advice not only on the emotional problems that can arise between two people for any number of reasons, but also on how to cope with the basics of living together, such as managing your finances and finding somewhere to live. The most successful relationships occur when partners have learned how to balance both the emotional and the practical aspects of their lives.

Within these pages you should find plenty of help and guidance for the road ahead, but the real key to a successful relationship lies in the amount of effort and compromise that each of you is prepared to put into your life together.

Couples who live together discover very quickly that their lives are not just linked emotionally. As soon as they start renting or buying property, or making formal provisions for each other, such as wills, they realise that there are also many financial and legal aspects to consider. The effects of some of these considerations will be much the same whether you are married or cohabiting. Others, however, demonstrate the ways in which the law views cohabiting differently from marriage and so are especially pertinent here. Some of these can have very significant effects, particularly if you later decide to break up or in the unfortunate event of one or other of you dying.

This book highlights many of the financial and legal implications of cohabiting, but it is not intended to be a detailed guide to finance or the law. The situation in regard to these matters is constantly changing and varies from country to country and even from state to state within a country such as the United States. For this reason, I recommend that you always seek professional advice if you are unsure of your rights or the meaning of any documents you are asked to sign, or if you have doubts about which course of action to take in a particular situation.

1

why do people live together?

Living together can simply be a matter of convenience. It is an excellent way of providing companionship, sharing costs and dealing with all the everyday necessities of life, such as putting a roof over your head, making meals and doing everyday chores. Most people who live together, however, choose to do so because they want, first and foremost, to set up home with and be with the person they love. They are driven by desire. The practical side of the relationship is often a secondary consideration in the rush to be together.

Generally, cohabitation is taken to mean a man and a woman living together as a couple without being married. In the UK, there is no legal definition of cohabitation, although it is possible to formalise certain aspects of the relationship by drawing up a cohabitation contract (see Legal Matters, starting on page 41). A solicitor can help you to do this. Such contracts are not yet enforceable in law in the UK, but they may at least serve to remind couples of their original commitment to each other. Contracts may also be drawn up for specific issues – for example, to indicate how each partner may benefit from the other's will or whether their home is owned jointly between them or by one person alone – and these are legally enforceable.

Contrary to popular belief, common law marriage does not exist in the eyes of the law in England. In Scotland, however, a cohabiting couple can be considered to have 'an irregular marriage by cohabitation and repute' if they are thought by friends and relatives to actually be married. A court can grant what is known as 'a declarator of marriage'. This then confers the same status on the couple that they would have if they were married.

The causes...

The reasons for living together can be many and varied. As I said earlier, it provides everything from love to someone to share the bills. For many people, however, living together is intended to be a prelude to marriage. In this case, it seems sensible to ask, why don't they just get married?

There are, it seems, several different reasons why not. Marriage, for many people, is a scary business. It can be an expensive undertaking both financially and emotionally. It is a very big step into the unknown and a very public statement of commitment. For those who are wary of taking this giant step, cohabiting is often regarded as a useful way of seeing how well they get on together. However, it has to be said that, although living together will test your compatibility with your partner in many ways, it is often not a very accurate 'dry run' for marriage because of the many differences between the two situations and the varying expectations people have of them.

Living together does share many similarities with marriage. For example, both married couples and those living together enjoy a relationship that is usually based on intimacy and trust, a sharing of resources and the wish for each partner to have a fulfilling role within the relationship. However, apart from the obvious legal differences between living together and marriage, studies have shown that there are many differences in the way couples tend to behave in cohabiting relationships, some of which I have listed below (obviously, these are generalisations and won't hold true in every case).

- In cohabitation, the relationship is more often one in which each partner is an equal. Cohabiting couples tend to share more of the traditionally 'gender specific' tasks such as shopping and cleaning than married couples.
- Couples who live together tend to keep their finances separate, often through separate bank accounts, even if they share many of the day-to-day costs of living together. Married couples usually pool their financial resources.
- If the female partner in a cohabiting couple has a greater income than the male, this tends to cause more friction than is the case in a marriage.
- Cohabiting couples with children in the home are more likely to separate than married couples with children at home.

It is certainly true that a great many people who start by living with someone have a fervent wish and expectation that the relationship will blossom into marriage. For such people, living together is often a good way of showing their loved one what a great catch they really are! For many others, however, living together is an end in itself and this may be for one of several reasons.

Living together may simply be the only option available to a couple who are unable or unwilling to marry but wish to spend their lives together.

Some people dislike what they regard as the institutionalised nature of marriage and the ritualised nature of the marriage ceremony itself. These people think that cohabiting is a convenient way for those who love each other to be together.

People whose parents were divorced may consider marriage to be a risky or even an emotionally painful experience. Many people who have themselves been married and divorced are often reluctant to marry again, especially if both partners in the new relationship have been divorced. Perhaps it is the fear of a second failure or the thought that in some way the pressures of actually being married contributed to the eventual divorce. Added to this, they may find it difficult to marry in church, and the thought of a registry office wedding may hold little appeal.

Some people live together because they feel that marriage is too constraining. They like the idea of sharing their life with a loved one but want the personal and financial freedom that cohabiting offers.

The broad categories of people who live together are usually determined by social or economic factors. But those who choose to live together rather than getting married also tend to fit particular personality profiles. For example, a large proportion of people who live together are self-employed or work on fixed contracts. They tend to have outside interests that do not involve their partner and which cause them to be away from the home for considerable periods of time. People who cohabit are not usually regular church-goers. They often live and work some distance away from their own family.

Couples aged 19 or less are the least likely to live together, but the largest numbers are found among 20 to 24-year-olds. There is a steady decline in percentages after that, with only about half as many people in the 40-to-45 age group cohabiting compared with those in the 19-to-24 age group.

9

...And the effects

Whatever the reasons for living together, one thing is not in doubt: if you and your partner decide to cohabit, it will be the start of a profound change in the type of relationship you have enjoyed up to now. A new chapter in your life will open and it is worth taking a moment to think about exactly what you are taking on. Statistics point to the fact that many cohabiting relationships are doomed to end in failure. Couples who live together before marriage divorce at a higher rate than those who do not. A survey in the United States found that a significant proportion of people in cohabiting relationships were less happy than those in traditional marriages.

There are no easy answers to explain why these findings are so, but it is often the case that people expect their live-in relationships somehow just to work automatically. They never do, of course. Unless you are that rare species, the perfectly matched couple, you must both be prepared to compromise, give and take, talk, listen, share and generally work pretty hard to make a success of things, especially in the early stages of a new relationship.

before you start

So you've decided to move in with your partner. It sounds like the perfect idea and you can't wait to put it into operation. But before you actually go ahead, take the time to stop and talk things over.

Talk to yourself

Examine your own motives and needs. At the outset, you should try to determine your goals and decide what you want to achieve personally from living with someone. Ask yourself a few questions.

What do I expect from this relationship?

Do you expect the cohabiting relationship with your partner will lead to marriage? Three out of four people living together say they expect eventually to get married – although the actual figure who do get married to each other turns out to be less in reality. Many sociologists also say that lots of couples cohabit because they do not believe that their relationship will endure – beware of self-fulfilment here! In any event, if the situation is not, in general, working out how you hoped or planned, you must be prepared to ask yourself, and your partner, how this situation can be changed.

Why did I choose this person?

The choices couples make when choosing marriage partners are often different from the choices we make when choosing someone as a live-in partner. Research suggests that a person's potential marriage partner usually tends to be similar to them in terms of their age, race and social background. These criteria are often less important when we choose a partner for living together, although cohabiters tend to have similar educational and employment backgrounds (perhaps not surprisingly when so many cohabiters meet initially through work.)

Is this leading to marriage?

If you definitely want your live-in partner to turn into a spouse in due course, here are some interesting pointers that may help you determine which way things are going to turn out.

- Females who have traditional values and strong kinship ties, especially with their parents, are usually more likely to be looking for marriage than females who do not.
- Females who are looking only to cohabit place a higher value on career and money than females who are looking to marry.
- Females looking to cohabit are more pessimistic about the chances of marriages succeeding and may have a history of family divorce.
- Males who are financially secure and have regular employment are usually more likely to want marriage than males who have insecure work patterns and non-traditional lifestyles.
- Males who have a history of family divorce, or who worry about divorce, are less likely marriage partners than males whose parents never divorced.
- Males who show little interest in having strong kinship ties usually turn out to be less likely to marry.

Are we compatible?

Even if eventual marriage isn't on the cards, everyone still wants their own living-together relationship to be romantic, fulfilling and enduring. Therefore it is important to try to assess how well your partner will fare as a long-term live-in prospect. To begin with, of course, you must be compatible with each other: you need to be sexually compatible, but it must go much deeper than that. If it's just lust, then the relationship is doomed to eventual failure.

Compatibility can be defined in several ways. Put in human terms, it means people getting along well together, but it essentially describes the state in which things exist together in harmony. To achieve compatibility, your relationship needs to comprise a number of different components, including friendship, respect and sexual attraction. The order in which they are described here is not significant. You just need to make sure they are there! As in many other aspects of living together, you'll find that many of these requirements are dependent on each other. You can't have one without the other.

Sexual attraction is probably what got you together with your partner in the first place. But even if sexual attraction only came about later, through getting to know each other, most couples wouldn't contemplate a live-in lifestyle without it. Being able to make each other feel good sexually, and wanting to do so, are vital ingredients of compatibility.

Friendship is a highly important aspect of living together. Most married couples and a good many live-in couples state that their partner is also their best friend. If you don't actually like the person you are living with (but only lust after him or her), then the relationship is unlikely to be going anywhere and you may as well resign yourself to the fact that it will finish when the lusting finishes. (Better still, you should have the courage to decide not to live together in the first place!) Real friendship is easy to recognise: you want to spend time with the other person, you find their company stimulating, and you want the best for them.

Respect and support are two more components of compatibility. Respecting someone means considering their feelings, needs and their point of view, as well as being faithful in the relationship. Supporting one's partner is something we sometimes take for granted, but it means more than just taking their side in arguments. It also means offering help when they are struggling with a problem and generally finding ways to make their life easier. Preventing someone from feeling stupid when they make a mistake is also a form of support and becomes automatic if you also respect someone.

Even with all of the above working in your favour, you need to be in harmony with your partner in other ways, too. It is important that you share the same values and share, or at least respect, each other's personal goals and ambitions. You should be in broad agreement about money matters and each other's work goals and also be at ease with your partner's friends and family since they are likely to feature quite a lot in your future life.

If you think you have all of the above qualities – at least in some measure – and can sustain them through the years ahead together, then you've probably got what it takes to make a compatible couple. Not only that, but you have also got love. And if you've got genuine love, that is the best ingredient for keeping any relationship together.

Talk to other people

Although it may seem that it is no one's business but yours and your partner's, your new situation will inevitably have effects on other people in all kinds of ways you had not envisaged. They, in turn, may treat you differently. So it is a good idea to talk your plans over with a few people close to you.

First there are your parents. These days, most parents don't try to talk their children out of living with someone, even if deep down they would rather see them married straight away instead. But both the expectation and the reality of failure in cohabiting relationships are high, and it is up to you to see that you make a success of your chosen lifestyle. (This probably does not apply when slightly older people decide to live together – somehow this is considered more normal and acceptable. Perhaps it's a case of 'They know what they are doing' or maybe it's because fewer children are born to unmarried parents in the older age groups.)

In some societies, there is still a religious or social stigma attached to living together, and if this applies to you, you may need to use tact and understanding to avoid hurting the feelings of parents and other loved ones when you tell them about your plans. And of course, whatever your beliefs and background, you clearly need to be at an age when you are legally allowed to cohabit.

It is almost inevitable when people live together that their social lives change in other ways, too. Some of the friends you each saw regularly when you were 'single' may figure less prominently once you are living together. There are several reasons for this – a change of location, different priorities, or the fact that you tend to socialise more with other couples now that you are together. It may even be because your partner just doesn't get on with some of your friends.

You will also need to consider your partner's immediate family, who are likely to figure much more in your social life than previously. Invitations to birthdays, Christmas and other celebrations that formerly only involved your partner will probably also include you now. You may not be very happy with this arrangement, but be prepared for it, nonetheless. It is almost certainly going to happen. Turning down invitations to join your partner and his or her family on these occasions is much harder when you live with someone, and refusing to do so will be likely to make you appear unsociable and unfriendly. It may give the impression that the two of you are not really an 'item' even though you live together. It also sends entirely the wrong message to your partner about his or her family and can be a source of ammunition in future arguments.

Talk to each other

It almost goes without saying that you and your partner should talk to each other before you take the final plunge and yet it is surprising how many people fail to do this. Take it from me, there are many things you should consider carefully and discuss together so that they do not cause friction once you are living under the same roof. The number of subjects ripe for argument is almost infinite, ranging from whether you intend to have children to who should pay the milkman. The time to sort them out is **now**, before you begin.

Where will you live?

One of your very first considerations will be thinking about, and then finding, somewhere to live. Now is the time to explore each other's views about the type of property you want and where you would like to live. Decide if you are going to rent – at least to begin with – or buy. Discuss the way you want to decorate and furnish the home and how much you can afford to pay.

Try to avoid overstretching yourselves financially. The very last thing you want is to be burdened with debts beyond your means at the start of a new relationship together. A big, expensive home is definitely not the best way to begin. A smaller but comfortable place that allows you to take stock of your new life and enables you some financial freedom is a far better option.

It is also worth remembering that buying or even renting a property will almost certainly have legal implications that will affect you both. If a property is jointly owned, you may both be legally responsible for maintaining payments on it. This also goes for other on-going financial commitments you may enter into jointly, such as the purchase of a car or furniture for the home, or the supply of other goods and services. Don't just assume that this will all sort itself out – talk about it **now**.

Who will pay for what?

While you may not necessarily wish to go into fine detail at this stage, it really is sensible to agree an outline of how you will manage your finances together, and who is going to pay for what. At the very least, it may make you realise that you are getting carried away and have miscalculated the cost of things. Before you move in together, try to discuss financial issues in an open manner. People sometimes feel mean or petty by talking about money issues, but they are essential elements of any marriage or cohabiting relationship. If you do not sort this out early, you risk the strong possibility that it will cause resentment later, which may damage your relationship. Should you split up at any time in the future, knowing how you shared out the costs will help to make it easier to sort out belongings and any outstanding payments to which you may both be committed.

As I said earlier, cohabiting relationships are viewed by some as more of a convenient partnership than marriages, with couples often remaining financially independent of each other. In many marriages, with incomes merged into a joint bank account, the issue of who pays for what is less relevant. In cohabiting arrangements, however, each partner's finances often remain independent so it is vital that you make it clear in advance how you are each going to contribute financially. It may sometimes be best to try to share all costs as equally as you can, taking into account any additional outgoings each of you may have (such as maintenance for an ex-wife and children), and making an allowance for salary or wage differentials. I shall talk about all this in detail later in the book.

Who will own what?

Ownership of property and goods can be complicated in living-together relationships, and it is a good idea to consider some ways of helping you to establish ownership of certain things. It will help to avoid later misunderstandings, and – although I hesitate to keep mentioning this at such an early stage – it will make matters much simpler in the event of your relationship breaking up. There are some simple general rules that apply, and I shall outline these in the chapter dealing with financial matters.

What about the children?

Quite often, people who decide to live together already have children from a previous relationship. Sometimes there are children from both partners' former relationships to be considered. There is no doubt that the presence of other people's children alters profoundly the nature of any relationship, so whatever the case, you must deal with this subject very early on. Do not underestimate the effects these small people may have on you, especially if they are not yours. You will need to accept them and be prepared to work hard to accommodate them into your life.

It may be that you are already well acquainted with your partner's children, so at least you may have had the opportunity to learn about their likes and dislikes, their moods and so on. Whether this is true or not, it is vitally important that you and your partner discuss how any children will affect your relationship. If you are a parent yourself, you will want to guarantee your children's happiness and will want to see them as often as you can. However, you must make special efforts to ensure that the relationship between your children and your new partner is also a happy one.

Think now about the effect your new relationship will have on the children themselves. If they are old enough to understand, the reasons you are going to live with someone should be explained to them, simply and clearly. Try to stress the positive aspects from their point of view and if there has been a break-up involving their parents, make it absolutely clear that they are in no way responsible for this.

Try to establish a few ground rules with your partner on how you deal with the children. You will want to make sure that you don't have arguments in front of them. Discuss your views on such matters as discipline, punishment and helping with household chores. The period before everyone is living under the same roof is the time to think through your own personal approach and strategy. And you should agree, whenever possible, to be consistent.

Think hard about your feelings towards your partner's children. Be prepared to discuss how you will deal with their feelings and manage any tricky situations (and there will be plenty of those). In the same way, think through your strategy if the children involved are yours. What are you going to do to help your partner's feelings? How are you going to make sure that no one feels left out or ignored? This is a real danger when only one partner has children – the childless partner may feel awkward and excluded, simply because everyone else is 'family', and may experience anxiety that they are losing their position in the household hierarchy. If this happens, it is vital that you talk it over together. The partner with the children will probably be unaware of the existence of the problem, because they are so bound up with trying to ensure the happiness of their offspring.

All of this will be all the more pertinent if the children are to live with you on a permanent basis. Apart from the sense of confusion and loneliness that the children may experience due to the separation of their parents, there is the likelihood of many other emotions manifesting themselves, ranging from resentment and jealousy towards your new partner to anger and outright hostility. You will have to be prepared to deal with all of this.

If you are the partner without children, you will have a different set of problems – dealing with and caring for someone else's children can be difficult at the best of times. It will often require a great deal of understanding, patience and lip-biting to get through the situations that will arise. You will have to realise that somehow a balance has to be achieved, or your partner may feel they are being forced to make a choice between their children and you.

It may be that the children will live more or less permanently with their other parent – particularly if this is their mother. This may mean that they then visit you at regular, pre-agreed intervals, such as on alternate weekends. You need to discuss how all of this is going to affect the children, you and your new partner.

Apart from the emotional issues, you must also consider the effect on your daily routine. What happens at holiday times? If your children live with you, do you need to live somewhere that will enable the children to continue their education at the same school? These are just a few of the many questions you must answer.

What about pets?

Less critical, but nonetheless still important, is the question of pets. You may 'inherit' a pet, because your partner has one already and where your partner goes, the pet goes, too. Fair enough, if you get along fine with this extra member of the household. But you need to work out a few ground rules between you. Whose pet is it now, especially when it makes a mess or needs feeding? Does it still belong to your partner, or are you now both responsible for it? Are you going to share the cost of keeping it? Are you going to look after it equally? How will you feel if your partner refers to your much-loved but aging pet as 'that mangy incontinent mutt'? On the whole, it makes for better feelings all round if the pet can be embraced by both partners as a welcome family addition and cared for equally by both.

On the other hand, if you are thinking of acquiring a pet to make the home complete, hold on! If you don't have to find a home for an animal straight away, it is best to wait a while. If the relationship between you doesn't work out, you won't want the added problem or even heartbreak of deciding what to do with an animal that it may no longer be possible to keep.

What about your social life?

Your social life may need to be reviewed. When you set up home with your partner, they may expect your leisure time to revolve more around the two of you being together – are you happy with that? Do you expect to carry on with pastimes and other activities that may not involve them? If so, how does your partner feel about this? If you are someone who normally enjoys several nights out a week with the boys (or the girls), is your partner going to happily accept this as a continuing situation once you are living together? Maybe you both still want to have time with your own friends. That's fine, if it suits you both, but make sure that it doesn't extend to the point when you spend more time out with your friends than with each other.

The key to success in any relationship, as we all know, is communication, and the more you and your partner talk about your hopes and feelings, the better. I should add that you will probably not agree on everything, but simply airing your views from the beginning means there is less chance of nasty surprises later on.

getting it together

So what is living together really going to be like? If you have never lived with anyone before, it can be strange at first always to have your partner around – but comforting and exciting, too. Most couples quickly settle into a pattern of living together that affords each of them the companionship, support and love they need, but which also allows both the 'space' to do the things they still want to do – read a book, watch an old movie on television or spend a few hours at a favourite pastime, for example. Don't crowd each other; you'll both still be there tomorrow! If one of you feels trapped or restricted in your new lifestyle, then it will cause resentment that may very quickly damage the relationship.

Quite often, when couples live together, one partner moves into the home of the other. You must try to remember from the outset that this is now a shared home. Even if you have been living in the home for some time without your partner, and have everything more or less as you like it, your partner may want to change certain things – the arrangement of the furniture or perhaps the décor. Again, compromise is the key. If you can't agree on everything (and few people do), then try to arrange things so that changes are not too abrupt to begin with. Alternatively, one of you could choose the colour schemes and decorations for the lounge, and the other could decide on the bedrooms, hallway and so on.

Key rules for living together

So, if we accept that everything is not going to be plain sailing from the word go, how do we avoid things becoming too rough? The answers, for the most part, are common sense but when feelings are running high that's often the first thing to go out of the window. Here are a few rules to bear in mind.

Be considerate

Being considerate means many things. It may mean agreeing to visit your partner's relatives when you would rather be doing something else. It certainly means not expecting your partner to clear up after you. It also means being proactive and thinking ahead sometimes. For example, if your partner is unexpectedly delayed for any reason and is likely to come home tired and hungry, fix a meal and have it waiting for them. In other words, being considerate means doing something to please your partner – even when it doesn't really suit you.

Learn to apologise

Say 'sorry' if it's your fault. This is never easy, because we seldom think things are our fault – it's always the other person that's wrong. But if you can both get into the habit of saying sorry, it can avoid the stand-offs, sullen glances and silences that often otherwise ensue.

Compromise

Be prepared to compromise with your partner. This is also partly about being considerate (see above). Most things in life, including many aspects of relationships, are a trade-off between what you really want and what you are prepared to give ground on to achieve more or less what you want. The compromises required when living together are many and varied. They can range from agreeing to take it in turns to choose the television viewing each night to deciding on a location for your home that suits you both in terms of travelling to work – even if it isn't perfect for either of you.

Share the boring jobs

Agree to share household chores. Is there really anyone who actually likes regularly doing housework or shopping for food? We would probably all rather have them done for us. However, someone has got to do these tasks, and the best way to avoid them becoming a burden is to share them – especially if you both work all day. If that is not always practical, at least divide all the different tasks equally so that the burden doesn't fall unreasonably on one person only.

There are several ways of doing this. One way is to simply take it in turns to do the weekly shopping and so on. An alternative way is to divide the tasks up so that you each do some. Whatever you agree, make sure you both stick to it.

Give each other personal space

Allow each other personal space. Although you are living together, it is quite natural for each of you to want to have some time for 'doing your own thing'. You don't need constantly to share every second doing things together – unless of course you have both said that is what you want.

Respect each other's belongings

Remember that private or personal possessions are just that – private and personal. You will jointly own, and share, many things in your new relationship, but there may be some things that are off limits to you. You will know what these items are, and everyone will have different ones. They could be diaries, photographs or other keepsakes. They could even be more seemingly mundane things; for example, you may think that a pair of delicate eyebrow tweezers from your partner's makeup bag makes a great tool for reaching an awkward screw on your car – but that view is unlikely to be shared so make sure you ask before you borrow them!

Mind your manners

Be friendly and polite to each other's friends and family. This sounds very obvious advice, but it is sometimes difficult to automatically accept other people's friends as your friends. However, give them the benefit of the doubt – after all, they can't be that bad if the one you love chose them as friends – and at least be as polite as you can until you get to know them. Try not to think of them as rivals for your partner's affections. The same goes for your partner's family. They are important to your partner, so try to get to know them quickly. Don't forget, your loved one's friends and family are going through the same process of acquaintance with you. The impression you give to them will affect how they feel about you in the future.

Don't take each other for granted

Remember that the reason you wanted to live together was because you wanted to spend as much time as possible with your partner. Do not start spending more time with your friends or simply pleasing yourself. Also, try not to fall into a routine in which your relationship becomes lazy. If your partner likes going out from time to time, make the effort for their sake. Don't assume that your partner is happy to do the things you are happy doing.

Communicate

This is one of the most important things that couples can do. Communicating isn't just about telling each other what sort of day you have had. Communicating can also help to ease worries about things that may be causing concern. You don't always have to speak in order to communicate; just a smile can convey all kinds of information. Communication can also prevent lots of arguments and resentment – so let your partner know if you are going to be in late, for example.

Don't have rows in public

Few things are more embarrassing or tedious than witnessing a couple having a public argument. These are often all the worse because the comments aimed at each other often seem petty or irrelevant to those forced to listen to them. Nothing is better designed to get you crossed off dinner party rounds than having a reputation for airing your disagreements in public. Hosts and hostesses like their gatherings to be fun and harmonious occasions, not a battleground for warring couples.

Don't embarrass your partner

This is perhaps an even greater sin than having a hearty row in public. It is very difficult to forgive someone for being made to feel small or in some other way inadequate in public. If you must make cutting or cruel remarks (and they are probably better left unsaid), save them for private consumption. But don't be surprised if you get a few choice observations in return!

Check your answerphone

No, that's not a mistake. Your recorded answerphone message may need altering since, ideally, it should now make it clear that you both live there. This may seem like a small issue perhaps, but this will help to reinforce the fact that you are an 'item' in the eyes of others. If you are moving into your partner's home, it will help you both to feel that this is now your home, too.

A word on personal habits

We have all got our own 'funny little ways' – we've lived with them all our lives and probably don't even realise they are in any way strange. However, your partner may not feel the same way when they are exposed to them on a daily basis, so be prepared to keep them to yourself or drop them altogether. You shouldn't try to become a totally different person, but you will both need to be more aware of each other's feelings about things such as tidiness and personal cleanliness. If possible, start trying to alter some of your potentially irritating ways before you set up home together. With luck, you may have ironed them out by the time you are under the same roof. If you are not sure if you actually have any annoying little foibles (but believe me, we all have), try asking someone close to you, such as a parent, brother or sister. They may not have actually mentioned them, but they'll know about them all right!

Take a look at this list of dos and don'ts – it will help you to recognise where your bad habits lie. Remember that for every one you can accuse your partner of, they will find two that you are guilty of.

Do:

- Clean up spills – especially if you caused them in the first place
- Replace the toilet roll if it is finished
- Hang up wet kitchen and bathroom towels
- Clean the bath or sink if you've left it in a mess
- Help clear up the kitchen after use
- Empty the dishwasher

- Make the bed if you got out of it last
- Turn the television down if your partner has gone to bed
- Flush the toilet and try to leave it smelling sweet – open the toilet window or use an air freshener if necessary
- Remember to add to the shopping list the item you've just used up.

Don't:

- Pick your nose or ears, EVER
- Cut your toenails anywhere but in the bathroom
- Leave the toilet seat up
- Start your meal before your partner is at the table
- Leave the table while your partner is still eating
- Help yourself to seconds without offering any to your partner
- Change television channels while your partner is watching something
- Read at the table – unless you are both reading the morning newspapers
- Leave all the dirty dishes to be washed or stacked in the dishwasher (and don't say you were going to do it later)
- Leave your personal items for your partner to clear up
- Strew your clothes everywhere so there is nowhere for your partner to sit
- Hang washing to dry over the bath when your partner wants to have a long comfortable soak
- Use the hairdryer if it interferes with the television picture
- Eat garlic, curry or anything strongly flavoured just before you go to bed

Of course, there are plenty more – you are probably aware of many of your partner's pet hates already – but if you can observe all of these, you are probably well on the road to laying the foundations for an enduring and happy relationship together.

Don't cut yourselves off

Once you are living together, normal life must go on. You need to remember that you still have responsibilities and other people to think of, apart from your partner. You must still be punctual for work, for example, even though you would probably rather stay luxuriating in bed with your new love. Sometimes people who live together become so bound up with each other that they forget that they have other friends and even family out there. Make plenty of time for each other, but make some time for other loved ones, too.

If your friends or family were unsure about you moving in together, there is no better antidote for allaying their fears than being invited to your new home so that they can see for themselves how natural and happy you both are together. You don't have to produce a banquet for them when they come round, either. Unless you are really keen to prepare a dinner party meal first time out, just invite them in for a drink and a few snacks.

There may be children in the relationship too, and it is important that they continue to receive the consideration they deserve. They need to feel that life is normal for them, and they will be more secure if there is a regular pattern to your home life. It is up to you to provide them with a happy and consistent environment, even if they are only weekend visitors.

4

financial matters

Since things change so quickly, the information in this chapter can only give you a broad guide. Laws and other regulations change regularly, and everyone's circumstances are different. Your local tax office and Inland Revenue department will be able to give you specific information and advice as it relates to you. You can also consult your bank, your accountant (if you have one) and other professional advisers for advice. Finally, the Citizens Advice Bureau provides an excellent source of help and information.

One of the key aspects of any close relationship, whether it is marriage or cohabiting, is finding the best way of handling your finances. In marriage, a couple's finances are often closely intermingled, even to the extent of sharing the same bank account. This is because married couples tend to demonstrate a stronger level of commitment at the start of their relationship than most cohabiting couples. It is also because they may each be setting up financial arrangements for the first time. Couples who decide to live together, on the other hand, may already have fairly well-established financial arrangements that they are reluctant to change (this illustrates one of the ways in which people who live together are more cautious about their relationship). This means that you have to take the time to sort out very carefully how you are going to handle your separate accounts and your joint outgoings.

Who pays for what?

There are several ways of deciding how to share the costs of living together.

Method 1: It doesn't matter who pays

The first way is for each of you to spend randomly. In other words, supermarket bills are simply paid by whoever is first at the checkout or by whichever partner happens to be on a shopping mission. If you are lucky, or if you have some sort of innate sense guiding you, it can work out over time that you both spend roughly the same amount of money. For this method to work in practice, of course, it requires you both to shop for the big purchases – like the weekly food shop – with the same sort of frequency. It may also mean one of you 'bankrolling' the other from time to time, because it is likely that there will be periods with this method when one or other partner is short of cash. It doesn't take a genius to work out that this method is fraught with problems and will almost certainly lead to rows unless, of course, you have so much money it really doesn't matter who spends what.

Method 2: We both pay equally

The second method is to share equally the cost of everything. This is certainly very simple: you just add up the cost of all of your purchases and outgoings and divide the total between you.

The drawback in this method is that if one partner is earning considerably more than the other, keeping up with the regular costs of running a house can sometimes cause a real financial strain on the lower-earning partner. This can then lead to hardship and even embarrassment when it comes to finding the funds to buy special gifts and so on. There are also added complications where one partner has financial commitments from a previous relationship – for example, maintenance payments as the result of a divorce settlement or dependent relatives. It is probably unreasonable to expect your new partner to help support your former spouse financially.

However, it does at least mean that if you decide to part, you know that you each have an equal call on the property you have bought between you.

Method 3: We both pay according to our income

The third way is an extension of the second method. You start by assuming that you will pay for everything jointly but take into account any major differences in salary or wage levels and adjust the shares accordingly. Make a further adjustment for any special financial commitments such as the ones alluded to above.

Method 4: We both pay for individual items in agreed proportions

A fourth way is to agree in advance what proportion of each bill you will each meet over a given period – this doesn't stop you from still sharing some costs equally if you wish and it takes into account any differences in your individual lifestyles. (For example, if your partner's parents live in Australia and he likes to phone them every week, you can adjust his share of the phone bill to reflect that.) You can draw up a table like the one below to help you plan your budget. What you decide to put on the list depends on your individual circumstances.

Expenditure	Full cost	His share	Her share
Mortgage/rent			
Gas/electricity			
Food			
Telephone			
Water			
Council tax			
Household insurances			
Household repairs			
Holidays			
Credit repayments			
Pet costs			
Car expenses			
Car fuel			
Family presents			
Total			

I have restricted my list to the items of expenditure that you are most likely to share, but you could, of course, also include clothing, personal items and any other outgoings on the list if you wished.

Creating a budget like this will also show how much your total expenditure will be over a given period of time. You will find more information about household budgets in Chapters 6 and 7.

In reality, how you determine what each of you spends can only be decided by agreeing on a system that is right for you both. However, I would recommend that, if you can, you do at least agree to share the payments for the rent or mortgage, the main bills, such as gas and electricity, and the cost of other major household items. This will help to foster a sense of partnership and equal commitment and prevents future arguments.

I have explained this system as it can be used for household running costs, but it can also be used for other items you buy. Remember that you should not only be in agreement about **how** you spend your money. It is also vitally important that you can agree on **what** you spend it on.

Organising payments

Once you have decided what each partner is going to contribute to the household budget, you must work out how to ensure the funds are there when they are needed to pay bills. First, you both need to get into the habit of considering this money to be already spent; it is no longer available to either of you as disposable income. You must put it to one side and only use it as you have decided.

One method of ensuring the money is saved is to open a separate account, to be used solely for paying any of these predetermined outgoings. Because the total bills may exceed your fund from time to time, it may be worth setting up a special account (often referred to as a 'budget account' or 'house management account') with your bank for this purpose. The money in this account can be added to each month by a direct debit from your normal account, and you can then use it to pay your regular bills or for any other outgoings that you have budgeted for. As long as you pay a regular amount into the account each month, and that the sum is equivalent to one-twelfth of your yearly outgoings, the bank will allow you to meet all your bills by providing an overdraft facility up to an agreed amount when necessary. All sorts of schemes for helping you to budget like this are available; talk to your bank, building society or other lender to find out about the best method for you.

One payment that will probably be deducted from your bank account at source is your regular mortgage payment, assuming you have bought a property. If this is the case, remember to include the cost of the mortgage payments (and indeed any other payments that may be already debited directly from your account) when calculating your total outgoings.

Some utility companies, as well as other organisations such as insurance companies, offer schemes whereby they deduct regularly an agreed amount from your bank account to meet the cost of their bills. It is worth considering all of these schemes, because they will make life simpler and they can sometimes save you money in the long term.

Accessing bank accounts

In certain circumstances, the position for cohabiting couples accessing their bank accounts is different from that of married couples.

When couples, married or not, have separate bank accounts, neither can access money held in the other's account. If one of a married couple with separate accounts dies, the bank may allow the other to withdraw the balance if the amount is small. In the case of a cohabiting couple, any monies in the account of a deceased partner will become the property of the estate and cannot be touched until the estate is settled.

If a married couple have a joint bank account, the money is owned jointly, regardless of who put the money into the account. If one partner dies, the whole amount becomes the property of the other. The same is true of a cohabiting couple with a joint account. If one partner should die, the other partner will be entitled to the balance and can continue to enjoy unlimited access to the account. Nevertheless, in this case, part of the money will be taken into account when it comes to evaluating the deceased partner's estate.

And a word on debt

As regards debts, each partner in a relationship, whether married or cohabiting, is liable for his or her own debts, and also for the whole of debts that are in joint names. I shall talk about this in more detail in the section on credit and borrowing (see page 39) and also in Chapter 6, Setting Up Home.

Being wise with your money

Today, there are more opportunities than ever for spending money. There are also many ways to save money, while still continuing to spend on the things you need. It is worth you and your partner taking some time to find the best ways to save on your joint outgoings.

Deregulation and opening up the market of many of the utilities (gas and electricity, for example) means that you can shop around to get the best deal. For instance, it may be cheaper for you to change your gas supplier, or to have one supplier provide you with both gas and electricity.

Banks, credit card companies and insurance companies bombard us daily with offers to open an account or take out a policy. Sometimes these can indeed save you money, and some are even tax efficient, but it is always worth getting as much information as possible before deciding. Similarly, some organisations encourage you to change your mortgage provider to save money or offer you a more flexible way of repaying your mortgage. Always ask about any penalties or administration charges involved in such schemes, however, before you sign anything. Seek professional advice from an independent source if you are unsure.

It is also worth considering taking out life assurance policies. These are designed to provide a sum of money to your loved ones in the event of your death, and you do not have to be married to benefit from them. Consult a reputable company or broker for information and advice.

If you have a mortgage, you are probably repaying the loan at a higher rate of interest than you receive from savings in, say, a building society account. With two of you now contributing to the household bills, it may be that you have some spare savings in a building society account. In this case it may be worth investigating with your mortgage lender whether or not you can use the savings to pay off part of the mortgage. For full details about mortgages, see page 60.

As I have mentioned several times above, it is well worth consulting a professional adviser if you find organising your finances difficult. Always choose one that is independent, i.e. not affiliated to any particular financial provider. They will be able to give you unbiased advice and help in choosing a savings scheme, insurance policy, mortgage, etc. that is right for you. Ask about their fees in advance – some may charge an hourly rate but many rely on the commission they receive for selling a scheme or policy to you.

Insurance policies

Nowadays you can take out insurance against almost anything. What you need will depend on your individual circumstances but I recommend that you consider all of the following.

- Buildings insurance – this is not usually necessary if you are renting from a landlord.
- House contents insurance – as well as your furniture and belongings, most policies will offer 'all risks' cover for personal items and cash, which you take out of the house. You should specify large expensive items such as computers and expensive pieces of furniture or jewellery.
- Life assurance – this will ensure that your dependants have something to live on if you die. You can also arrange a policy to provide extra money when you retire.
- Car insurance – you must, by law, have at least third party insurance for your car. For an additional charge you can be protected against theft, fire and damage. If you buy a new car, you may also want to take out an extended warranty after the manufacturer's warranty has expired.
- Long-term sickness insurance – this will guarantee you an income if you are ill and unable to work for months at a time.
- Private health insurance.
- Pet insurance – this can provide cover against the cost of vet's bills and also in case your pet causes damage to another person or their property.

Be sure to read the fine print of all insurance policies – whether they be for property, home contents, life, car or whatever. Some life assurance policies may have restrictions on who benefits. It could be that although a spouse is a beneficiary, a live-in partner may not be. Look out for other kinds of restrictions too. For example, your property insurance may not cover for certain kinds of damage – these clauses are known as exclusions. There may also be the possibility of your premium increasing if you make a claim. Many policies insist that you pay a proportion towards any claim (known as the excess).

It is important to check these details closely, especially if your circumstances change through divorce or cohabitation, for example. If in doubt, ask your insurance company or broker to explain any specific details of the policy that are not clear to you. Like many other goods and services, you can often find a better deal on insurance policies by shopping around for quotations. Be sure to ascertain if there are any penalties for changing a policy – some companies charge an administration fee for making alterations, or cancelling or setting up a new policy.

Taxation

In the UK, all couples living together are taxed separately and each partner automatically receives a single person's allowance. There is still an allowance for married couples, but it only applies to couples where one person was born before 6 April 1935, so for most couples there is no tax advantage or disadvantage in not marrying.

Tax allowances for children have now been replaced by the children's tax credit, which, in the case of separated or divorced parents, may be claimed by the parent with whom the child lives. You or your partner may also be eligible for the working families' tax credit. Tax credits are not given automatically – you must apply for them. Forms are available from your local tax office.

It is worth checking your eligibility for tax allowances and credits every year as the system is very complicated and subject to changes on an annual basis. You can obtain help and advice on all the above from your local tax office or by telephoning the Inland Revenue helpline on 0845 300 1036.

Benefits

Heterosexual partners, whether cohabiting or married, are assessed in the same way for entitlement to benefits such as income support, income-based jobseeker's allowance and housing benefit. They are treated as a couple and their income is assessed jointly. This situation does not apply for gay and lesbian couples, however. Contact your local Benefits Agency office for full details.

Your entitlement to most national insurance contributory benefits is determined by your contribution record. It is not possible for you to get an increase for an adult dependant if you are not married to her or him, except where that partner is caring for children.

Student loans

If you are applying for a student loan, your partner's income will usually be taken into consideration when assessing your eligibility. There are exceptions, so contact your Local Education Authority for full details.

Pensions

Cohabiting partners cannot claim a spouse's retirement pension or a widow's pension paid by the state. The situation regarding occupational and personal pension schemes will depend on the rules of the particular scheme. At the moment, all occupational pension schemes must offer equal benefits to husbands and wives and most schemes offer benefits to dependent children and some will extend this to a dependent heterosexual partner. Few, however, will offer benefits to lesbian or homosexual partners.

If you and your partner wish to prepare a personal pension scheme to cover your old age, this can be done even though you are not married. A scheme can be set up to provide cover to whoever the pension scheme member decides, as long as the pension scheme member pays the necessary contributions to the fund. If you wish to do this, contact an independent financial adviser.

Credit and borrowing

For most people, as we have seen, the biggest single loan they will require will be for the purchase of a home. However, there may be many other things you need that are beyond your day-to-day finances to buy them outright. These can include the purchase of a car, holidays, home improvements and home repairs. When such expenses loom, you will probably need either to enter into a contract to purchase the goods by instalments or to borrow some money to buy the goods for cash.

Goods that are purchased can normally be bought on hire purchase or credit terms. You may be required to pay a deposit, after which you can take the goods. You are then required to pay an agreed amount – usually monthly – until the debt is cleared and the goods become your property. Usually, the price you pay for goods in this way is higher than the cost would be if purchased outright for cash. The difference between the two prices is the interest – a profit made on the loan, which you pay. Some purchase agreements offer interest-free credit, so that you simply pay back the actual cost of the goods over time. This type of offer is usually well advertised at the time you buy.

If there is interest to be paid on the loan, you can quite easily calculate how much this will be; in many cases it will be stated somewhere on the agreement. Before deciding to accept the contract, it may be worth seeing if it is cheaper for you to buy the goods for cash by borrowing the money. Of course, you will still be required to pay back the cash loan, but the rate may be cheaper. It pays to shop around. Banks, building societies and other money lending institutions will all have information about their rates for borrowers. Some of the best deals can be had by going online. If you do not have a computer, you can still access the information by using the internet facilities in internet cafés or some public libraries.

Some services, such as house repairs, will usually be carried out by companies or individuals who will expect to be paid in full when the job is done; indeed, some may even expect to be paid as work progresses. In these instances, a cash loan is probably the only option available to you.

Be sure when entering into any such agreements, which are normally legally binding, that you have the resources to pay the instalments – remember, these will need to be added to your budget.

A word on credit payments (or lack of them): if your partner runs off leaving you with goods that are still subject to hire purchase or credit payments, but are in their name only, you should not be held liable for the payments. However, it is advisable to write to the company or organisation whose goods are involved, explaining the situation and inviting their collection – or offering to carry on with the payments yourself if you want to keep the goods. It will be up to the company concerned to decide which course of action they wish to follow.

If the credit agreement is in both cohabiting partners' names, the owners of the goods have the right to enforce payment from either or both partners, or to repossess the goods if payment is not made. Alternatively, you may be able to continue to pay the amount alone, in certain circumstances.

5

legal matters

Many aspects of living together involve some kind of legal contract. This is frequently the case with financial obligations, for example when buying property or other goods. There are also the legal implications of renting and the various rights each partner will have within the law regarding their option to remain in the home following a break-up, for example.

Housing and the law

The cohabiting partner of a tenant, in either public sector or private accommodation, has no rights to remain in the home if the tenant withdraws permission for him or her to stay. (This contrasts with the situation regarding married couples, in which both spouses have a right to remain in the home unless a court order decrees otherwise.) The cohabiting partner can apply to a court to get a short-term right to stay, however. In Scotland, it may be possible to prove joint tenancy anyway, if both partners moved into the home at the same time.

It is advisable, therefore, to have the tenancy agreement drawn up so that you and your partner are joint tenants. This gives you equal rights, but it also gives you equal responsibilities in the event of rent arrears and so on. Sole tenancies can be converted to joint tenancies with the landlord's permission. So if, for instance, you move into a property already rented by your partner, you could arrange for the tenancy to be put in both of your names.

If a sole tenant should die, the surviving heterosexual partner can usually take on the tenancy. It is also sometimes permissible for surviving lesbian and gay partners to succeed to the tenancy in public sector accommodation.

If the property is owned by only one partner, the other cohabiting partner may have rights to remain in the home if it can be proved that he or she contributed towards the purchase and upkeep of the property. However, if the threat of eviction occurs, it is advisable to seek professional legal advice because it may be possible to avoid this happening.

If there are children in the relationship, a court may decide to include property as part of the overall settlement to help ensure the protection of the children in the event of a break-up.

Ownership of property

There are considerable differences in the way the law views married couples and cohabiting couples, and none more so than in the case of property. In the event of the divorce of a married couple, it is usually assumed that everything the couple has is owned jointly, regardless of who actually paid for it at the time it was purchased. Therefore, as part of the divorce proceedings, a court will ensure, if necessary, that the assets of the previous marriage are divided equitably, taking into account any special circumstances such as the continuing care and financial support of children resulting from the marriage.

Since the status of living together is not recognised in the same way in law, it does not follow, should you and your partner break up, that all of your assets will be divided fairly or equally between you. So, for example, unless your home is owned in both your names, only the person whose name appears on the deeds will be entitled to the proceeds of the sale of the property, even if both partners have paid equally towards its purchase. This is why it is essential that you consider putting all major financial commitments, such as the purchase of your home, in joint names.

The same advice goes for other large purchases such as cars and furniture. It is one thing to assume, at the start of what looks like becoming a loving, permanent relationship, that you will agree on a fair sharing-out of assets should you break up. After all, you just cannot imagine it ever happening. However, it is a sad but very true fact that a high percentage of cohabiting couples do break up, just as married couples do. During the painful and acrimonious atmosphere that often prevails during parting, it is a plain fact of human nature that people are not always at their most generous and fair-minded.

There are a few general rules that do apply. For example, any property owned by one or other partner before he or she began cohabiting remains his or her property. Any items bought by one person remains his or her property. It is considered to be jointly owned if it was purchased from a joint account, however. Anything given by one partner to the other belongs to the recipient – although technically this can be difficult to prove. If one partner gives the other housekeeping money, any items bought with it will probably be considered to be the property of the person giving the money.

Despite the above, unless you have some form of contract or documentation to prove joint ownership of items, you may find that you have a real battle on your hands to ensure a satisfactory split of such assets. You can quite easily create a list, of which you each have a copy, stating that the items on it are jointly owned and will, in the event of your relationship ending, be divided equally between you. It is then simply a matter of adding any such items to each list and both of you signing or initialling each item as it is added. It may be also be useful to add next to each item its value.

If one of you is paying for most of the things, this may not be the best solution. Instead, you can simply write the name of the purchaser against each item, designating that person as the owner.

Cohabitation agreements

You can, of course, go a step further and draw up a complete cohabitation agreement. Ideally, this should be a non-threatening, mutually agreed document, signed by each party – a sort of contract between couples who live together. In Britain, at the present time, cohabitation agreements may be difficult to enforce legally, but they can at least set out in writing what your intentions are regarding the joint ownership of various assets, for instance. In the event of a break-up, a court would have the evidence of your intentions to help it make a decision. If you wish to draw up a cohabitation agreement, you should both seek the advice of a solicitor.

In America, cohabitation agreements are more commonplace, because they are recognised as the basis upon which to claim legal compensation in certain situations. Even there, however, they are not enforceable in all states.

Even when cohabitation agreements are recognised, there are certain rights that are, by law, restricted to spouses. No matter how long your cohabiting relationship may be, the following will apply:

41

- You will not automatically inherit your partner's assets in the event of their death.
- You cannot claim your partner's social security benefits.
- You may not expect entitlement to private health care and other benefits that your partner may enjoy as part of his or her company benefits package.
- You and your partner cannot transfer assets to each other without paying tax.
- You cannot assert the right not to testify against your partner in a law court.
- You cannot assert legal jurisdiction over your partner if he or she becomes unable to handle his or her affairs.

Despite these fairly considerable caveats, a cohabitation agreement can provide lots of other benefits. These include the clarification of each partner's financial position, details about jointly accrued property, responsibilities for leases, inheritances and so on. You should consult a solicitor or other legal adviser about all these details.

If you do decide to draw up a cohabitation agreement, I would recommend that it should cover arrangements for the following, both present and in the event of the death of one partner or the end of the relationship:

- The ownership of major items
- The distribution of property and other items
- Arrangements and financial obligations for children
- Arrangements for pets
- Settlements of joint leases and debts

Making a will

As I mentioned above, in a cohabiting relationship, if one of you should die without leaving a will (this is known as being intestate), the surviving partner will not automatically inherit anything unless it was owned jointly. Therefore it is vital that you both make wills to ensure your partner inherits in the event of a death. Again, this is different from the situation in a marriage, where the surviving spouse will normally automatically inherit some or all of the estate (the goods and property of the deceased).

A will allows you to decide who should benefit from your goods, and in what proportion. You may think that the whole process is a bit unnecessary, but if you do not make a will, your property and all your assets may be divided up in a way that would not please you. For example, if you are divorced with children and you have not made a will, the courts could decide that your ex-spouse should benefit in the event of your death. This could cause great financial hardship to your present partner, who could even lose your shared home as a result. If you die intestate and you have no blood relatives, your property will go to the Crown. If you have children from your relationship, you may want to appoint a guardian to care for them after your death. There are also tax-efficient advantages to making a will (you should seek specialist legal advice on this). You will probably agree, then, that it is worth taking the time and trouble to make a will.

In Britain, you must be at least 18 years old to make a will, and it must be written or typed and signed in front of the appropriate witnesses (usually at least two) who must also sign the will in your presence. If you have assigned part or all of your goods to your partner, he or she must not then be a signatory to the will. There are certain restrictions on the types of property that can pass to others under a will, including certain insurance policy funds and pension schemes. For this reason, when taking out such policies, you might wish to consider taking out policies that specifically name your partner as the beneficiary (the one who benefits). Alternatively, you may wish to enquire as to the possibility of changing existing policies to include your partner. You should seek professional advice from independent brokers to ensure you have the necessary cover.

When you make a will, it is usual to appoint someone to manage the distribution of your goods or property. Such a person, or persons, is called an executor. There are packs available to enable you to draw up a will by yourself if you feel competent. However, a solicitor will handle all the details for you instead if you prefer.

Other issues

There are a few other areas where the law's view of cohabiting couples is different from its view of married couples.

In both civil and criminal court proceedings, cohabiting partners are treated as though they have no relationship to each other.

Cohabiting couples cannot legally adopt a child and, unlike married couples, they can act or testify against each other in court.

However, if there is ever any domestic violence in a relationship, the situation is the same as it would be for married couples: a cohabiting partner can apply for a court order for protection against his or her partner. This may result in the violent partner being ordered to leave the home for a defined period. The violent partner may face arrest if he or she does not comply with the court order.

A woman in a cohabiting relationship can take decisions regarding contraception and abortion without first needing to ask her partner, and either can decide to be sterilised without getting the other's consent. In marriage, a husband's consent is not legally required, but some doctors and clinics may ask for this before performing a sterilisation or abortion, and even before fitting a contraceptive coil. They may also ask for a wife's consent before sterilising her husband.

In some circumstances, for example when going into hospital or filling in life insurance forms, you may be asked to provide the name of your next of kin. This is usually taken to describe your nearest relative, by blood, by adoption or by marriage. Your cohabiting partner therefore does not qualify as your next of kin, and cannot be entered as such.

6

setting up home

It may be that one (or both) of you already owns a home. In this case, you can choose either to move into the accommodation already occupied by one of you, or start looking for a new place.

Choosing your first home together with your partner should be fun – and it can be. But, unfortunately, looking for and securing the right property can also be a stressful and time-consuming business. Try not to let it get you down if your efforts come to nothing at the start. If you persevere, and use the information here, eventually you will find the right place for both of you.

What sort of home?

If you are starting afresh, you will have to make a number of key decisions. Now, if not before, is the time to start thinking 'We'. The type of property you decide to live in, where it is and how you finance it, should be joint decisions. Some things you may have little control over, such as how much you can afford, but where there is a choice be sure you both want, or at least agree on, the same thing by asking yourselves a few questions.

- What sort of home are you looking for – flat, maisonette or house?
- How many rooms do you need? (Don't forget, you may want room for guests.)
- Do you need a property that will allow you to expand your options – can you use it as a work-from-home office, for example?
- What area are you going to look in? Are you going to decide equally where you both live or is one of you going to have to make compromises?
- How much can you afford to spend?
- How are you going to pay for the home – rent or purchase?

- If you rent, how long will the lease be for?
- Will the leasing agreement or mortgage (if you decide to buy) be in one partner's name or in joint names?
- What furniture and other items are you each bringing to the property, and what will you need to obtain?

To a large degree, whether you choose a flat or a house is a choice you must make based upon your finances and your personal preferences. Most couples cohabiting for the first time choose a flat. The reasons are easy to see. Flats are usually more affordable and more abundant. There is less maintenance and often no garden to keep tidy and fewer furnishings are required. When you want time for each other, you don't need an overgrown lawn for competition!

On the downside, flats can sometimes be a bit noisy, because you are surrounded by other tenants, and they don't always offer the privacy of a house or maisonette. There is less storage space and sometimes nowhere really suitable to park the car. Unloading the shopping can also be an inconvenience – particularly if you live at the top of a block of flats with no lift.

Maisonettes are a sort of halfway stage between a flat and a house. They usually have their own front door at street level and are completely self-contained. They usually comprise either the top floor or the bottom floor of a two-storey house. They can offer many of the advantages of a small house without all the costs often associated with a house. You may have other occupants living directly above, or below you, so noise can still be a potential problem.

A house is often the preferred choice of couples who have already cohabited for some time and couples with more substantial funds available. Couples with children from one or both partners' former relationships may prefer a house because this gives them more space and possibly separate bedrooms for the children. It is more likely that a house will have space to park a car outside, on the driveway or in a garage. This is an important consideration if both you and your partner have cars – which is more often the case than with newly married couples.

Apart from the inevitably higher costs associated with running a house compared with a flat or maisonette, there is usually more general housekeeping and maintenance required, too. However, the extra space and privacy, as well as the enjoyment derived from a garden, usually outweigh any other considerations.

Location

Once you have decided on the type of accommodation that's right for you, you must decide on a location. This may sound easy, but there are often many factors to consider. First, do you both work, and if so, is the location suitable for each of you to commute? Some compromising may be inevitable. Are you prepared for the possibility of one of you being asked to relocate somewhere entirely different as a result of your work?

If you have children from previous relationships who are still living more or less permanently with your previous spouse or partner, how close to them is your new place going to be? You may need to choose somewhere more or less equidistant if you and your new partner both have children to consider in this way. It is more reassuring for children to know that you are not living very far away. Sometimes you cannot avoid moving some distance from your children, and your previous partner may move away with them in any case. However, the more often it is possible to see your children, and the closer you are to them geographically, the better.

How much to spend?

Everyone's circumstances are different, and the actual amount you decide to spend on renting or buying a property will depend on your budget – your income and your outgoings. If you are taking out a loan to buy a property, your loan will be calculated on the basis of your salaries or wages. Many people overstretch themselves, both when borrowing money to buy a property and when deciding how much rent they can afford. It's human nature always to want what is slightly beyond one's price range! However, you should try to resist the temptation to overspend; other costs and outgoings always seem to be greater than you first imagined, and the last thing any newly cohabiting couple need is an argument over money.

Do take a cool, realistic look at your financial situation before committing yourselves. If one of you is self-employed, how regular is your income? Earnings for self-employed people can fluctuate, and this should be taken into account when budgeting. If you are seeking a mortgage or other loan, you may be required to show documentary evidence of a steady level of income (ideally, a set of properly audited accounts) for a number of years as a self-employed person before a loan is granted. Before deciding how much you can afford, reread the chapter entitled Financial Matters.

Renting

Many people begin living together by renting a property. Another case of 'wait and see' perhaps, but it is also often the quickest way of getting together under the same roof when starting out. Renting, rather than buying, can also give you more flexibility. For example, if you want to move out quickly, you can do so provided you have given due notice and paid for the period of your agreement. There is no property to be sold first before moving. Renting may also tie up less of your money, although most tenancy agreements include a security deposit, which must be paid at the start of the tenancy, and the monthly rental on some properties can exceed the monthly repayments of a mortgage. You should remember that no matter how low the monthly payments are, they are going into someone else's pocket. If you were paying the same amount into a mortgage scheme, you would at least have something to show for it in the long term.

Other disadvantages of rented accommodation include the fact that you never enjoy the feeling of owning your very own place, and it can sometimes be difficult to obtain permission to redecorate it to your own personal taste. Even if you are allowed to make improvements to the property, you are unlikely to reap the financial benefits when you decide to move out – although your landlord will!

You will usually be expected to enter into a contractual agreement when you rent a property. This will involve you providing certain personal and financial details to enable the landlord or agent to determine your suitability to rent the property. It is important to be truthful when providing this information, otherwise you could invalidate your tenancy. You will also be expected to agree to certain conditions. For example, the agreement may stipulate that no pets are allowed on the property. Although tenants in rented properties usually have the same broad legal rights throughout a particular country, the contractual details of rented accommodation vary in the UK, and the terms and conditions in one property will not necessarily be exactly the same in another. You may also be expected to pay a deposit.

Rented property must be kept in good condition by the tenant, but some contracts provide a cleaning and even a gardening service as part of the agreement. Although you will usually be expected to pay for all the gas and electricity consumed, you may find that you are not charged for things like water rates, etc. If the full terms are not stated on your contract, be sure to enquire.

Many rented flats and houses have restrictions on children, as well as the keeping of pets mentioned above – and even on the playing of ball games and other activities. Violating these restrictions could jeopardise your tenancy agreement. If you have children or pets, such properties may clearly be unsuitable for you. It is best to find out about any such caveats right at the start, therefore, before you sign anything.

There are several ways to go about finding private rented accommodation. Letting agents, including the rented property sections of many estate agents, advertisements in local papers and specialist publications, the internet and even shop windows are all worth investigating. Good properties usually go very quickly, however, so get yourself on mailing lists and be prepared to spend plenty of time on the telephone or the computer. Don't simply wait for estate agents and others to ring you or mail you with details, but make a point of calling them on a regular basis in case something has just become available.

Accommodation agencies are often able to find accommodation for people looking for private sector housing. If you register with such an agency they will ask for details about the kind of property you want and how much you want to pay. They will usually also need details about your job and income. You may be asked to provide references from your employer, present or previous landlord and bank. An accommodation agency can decline to register you on its books. It is not against the law in the UK for it to do this.

If you register with an accommodation agency in the UK, the agency should only charge you a fee if it finds you somewhere to live. It is illegal for an agency to charge for putting your name on its list or for simply taking details. It is also against the law for the agency to request payment for providing a list of properties available to rent. Furthermore, the agency should not charge a deposit that it promises to return if no suitable accommodation is found.

If you are offered accommodation, always be sure that you and your partner both inspect the property and satisfy yourselves about all the terms and conditions of the tenancy agreement before accepting it. (The terms and conditions can include the amount of rent, whether or not there is a security deposit, and whether or not there is a mortgage on the property – if there is, you could be evicted if the landlord defaults on the mortgage payments.) It is up to you to make certain that you understand fully the terms of any contract before you sign. If you are unsure, ask questions, or enlist the help of a solicitor or other professional adviser to help you first.

Tenancy agreements

When you rent a property, it is usual to sign a tenancy agreement. The agreement gives both you and the landlord certain rights. For example, it gives you the right to inhabit the property and the landlord the right to receive rent from you. In England and Wales, most tenants do not have a legal right to a written tenancy agreement, but local authorities and housing associations will provide written agreements. In Scotland, the landlord must usually provide a written tenancy agreement. Even an oral tenancy agreement is, nevertheless, a legal agreement, although it may be difficult to enforce in law if nothing is put down in writing.

There are different sorts of contractual arrangements, and you should be aware of the effects of the contract you and/or your partner sign. The best advice is perhaps that you should decide in advance what you and your partner want in the way of contractual obligations and then see if the landlord will agree to your terms. It must be said, however, that most landlords will simply insist on the terms they already have in place. Some agencies insist that both partners leasing a property sign the agreement and others may be happy for there to be only one signatory. Joint signatures imply joint rights and responsibilities. So, if you have shared the deposit, you should probably both sign. Your signature will ensure that you will have access to the property if your partner leaves you, but it will also bind you to the contract – and any payments due.

You may sign a joint or sole tenancy agreement. In the case of joint tenancy, each tenant has an equal right to remain in the property and not to be excluded without a court order. Each is legally liable for the whole rent and can be pursued for the whole amount. Each tenant has equal rights to apply for housing benefit for his or her share of the rent. If one joint tenant dies, the other automatically inherits the whole tenancy. As long as one joint tenant occupies the property, housing status security rights are protected. Thus if one partner leaves, the other is entitled to remain in the property. Overall, then, under a joint tenancy arrangement, there is considerable protection for both partners against eviction.

Under a sole tenancy agreement, only the tenant who signs the contract has the right to occupy the property under housing law. This means if your partner is the sole tenant, they can evict you! On the other hand, they have the responsibility for paying the rent to the landlord. If a sole tenant dies, anyone else occupying the property will usually have to move out. Any agreement between the sole tenant and other occupants is strictly between them. The other occupants have no agreement with the landlord.

For maximum protection, any kind of written tenancy agreement should be signed by both parties and each should have a copy. The agreement should include:

- The names of both the landlord and the tenants (you, of course, are the tenants)
- The address of the property
- The date the tenancy starts and its duration
- Who else, if anyone, is allowed to use the property
- The details of the rent, including when it is to be paid
- Whether any services are included by the landlord (such as gardening) and if there is a charge for these
- The notice period to be given by either party in the case of termination of the agreement

There are numerous clauses and conditions relating to tenancy agreements. By law, in the UK, you should receive a rent book if your tenancy is weekly. The landlord must also provide you with his or her address. Changes to a tenancy agreement can normally only be implemented if both parties agree to them. If this is the case, then a new agreement should be drawn up or the changes documented in writing.

There are also certain rights that are implicit in tenancy agreements. These include the right of the tenant to have basic repairs (such as mending a leaking roof) carried out by the landlord, to have the installations for the supplies of water, sanitation, electricity and/or gas to be kept in good working condition, and the right to live peacefully in the property without the landlord causing a nuisance.

Deposits and key money

The landlord may ask you, his tenants, to pay a holding deposit and a security deposit. The holding deposit is used to secure the property on your behalf until you have signed the contract. Once the holding deposit is paid, it is usually non-returnable except in particular circumstances – such as the accommodation not being ready for you to move into on the agreed date. Do not expect to get a holding deposit back just because you have been offered a more suitable property!

The security deposit covers the landlord against default on the part of the tenant. It may also be used to cover the cost of repairing the property against any damage that you cause; when your agreement is terminated, you may find some of your deposit being withheld to cover the cost of cleaning the carpets, for example. If the amount withheld is for a specific reason, such as carpet cleaning just described, you should satisfy yourself that the money deducted is a reasonable and fair amount.

The landlord may also charge you key money for giving you the tenancy of a property. If the sum being asked seems unreasonable, your only course of action is to refuse the property. Make sure you are aware of this possible cost, and the amount, before you sign anything.

Public sector accommodation

Normally, people who want local authority housing must apply to go on a waiting list first. Various circumstances are taken into account when determining the housing priority of applicants and certain conditions must be satisfied if you are to be considered eligible. Contact the housing department of your local council for details. The local authority will generally house homeless families with children, after a stay in emergency or temporary accommodation. Single people and couples without children may be allowed to stay in emergency accommodation initially, but are then likely to have to seek private sector rented accommodation.

The only way to ensure that you will get permanent accommodation from a local authority in England and Wales is to have yourself placed on their registered list. You may not be eligible to go on such a waiting list if you have recently arrived in or returned to the UK. In Scotland, anyone over the age of 16 can apply to go on the waiting list, but again, this does not automatically mean you are eligible for accommodation. Different authorities employ different methods to determine priority to applicants. Most commonly, a points system is used; the higher your number of points, the more likely you are to be offered accommodation. Points are awarded according to your length of time on the waiting list, age, length of residence in the area, condition of health, number of family members and their ability to remain together in existing accommodation.

The Citizens Advice Bureau will give advice and help you to process your application.

Sometimes the local authority and local registered social landlords – for example, housing associations – operate a joint register. An applicant can, in these circumstances, register for both types of housing by filling in a single form. Otherwise, a person wishing to be considered for housing association accommodation must be nominated by the local authority.

If you are looking for this type of accommodation, it will be useful to obtain lists of local accommodation agencies, housing associations and cooperatives as well as contacting the local authority.

Buying

Many couples start off by renting accommodation together, to see how things work out between them. In time, if the relationship between them develops well, and if finances permit, they may decide to buy somewhere together. Not only does buying a property give you the added security of permanent accommodation if you so desire, it also sends a pleasant signal to each of you that you are thinking long-term about the relationship.

Buying a property is exciting but becoming an owner–occupier is a huge financial undertaking for most people – probably the biggest single cost they will ever incur – and it should be considered carefully before you decide to do it. Although the values of properties usually rise, enabling you to make a profit when you sell, if you have to sell quickly for any reason, or at the wrong time, you may find that you are out of pocket. There are also a lot of ancillary costs associated with purchasing a house (see later), which can take some time to recoup.

New or old?

If you are buying a property, one consideration will be whether to buy a new or an older place. There are advantages and disadvantages to both choices.

A brand-new property will reduce the links in the selling 'chain' that can be so much a feature of property buying. If you have no property of your own to sell, you can move into a new place as soon as it is built. Because it is new, the property will not require any repairs or modifications before you can secure your loan on it or are able to move in.

New properties are usually covered by a guarantee that protects the owners against the cost of major structural repairs for a number of years. When a new property is being built, there is often the opportunity for the buyer to choose the style of tiling, bathroom and kitchen fittings and other accessories that will be used in its construction.

New houses in the UK are designed to be economical to live in. They usually feature double glazing on the windows and doors, low-maintenance soffits and fascias and good levels of loft insulation. Some have cavity wall insulation. All these things help to reduce costs by cutting maintenance and heating bills. They also help to maintain or enhance the value of the property should you want to sell it in the future.

A few years ago, the accusation levelled against many new properties was that they had a uniform, box-like appearance with little real style. Today, however, many new houses incorporate attractive brickwork, windows and other features, helping to make them highly individual abodes. Many of these features – such as a variety of different brick styles being used in the construction – are copied from those found on older buildings.

Set against all of these advantages is the fact that new houses can appear quite expensive and there is usually less opportunity to negotiate a price reduction – although this depends, to some extent, on demand. Because the builder may attempt to obtain planning permission to build as many units as possible on a site, the gardens are also often small and the buildings are packed close together. Another problem that can be associated with new houses is a lack of a real sense of exactly how a development, or even an individual house, will finally look when it is finished. Plans are often modified during the construction of a development, leading to disappointment on the part of some buyers with the final outcome. Be wary of lush green fields adjacent to your development – the chances are that some developer has them in mind as a future site for more properties.

So what about an old property? Many of the advantages of a new property become disadvantages with an old property, and vice versa. Thus, to begin with, you may be subject to the selling chain when buying an older place. Older houses and flats may need repairs before you can move in, and they will probably need more general maintenance due to their age.

Old properties can be draughty due to badly fitting windows and doors – unless previous owners have fitted modern replacement windows and doors. House building regulations often specify the amount of loft insulation and so on to be installed in new properties, but older houses may have much less – or even none at all. In this case, you will need to add this to keep fuel costs low.

Someone else's idea of decoration may not be the same as yours, and it is likely that you will need to spend more time and effort redecorating an older property to turn it into your dream home. However, this can also be a rewarding task, and many a fine fireplace or beautiful set of wooden banisters has been rediscovered from beneath previous layers of 'modern' decoration by a new owner renovating an old property.

One of the reasons many people decide on an old property is because it has 'character'. A builder can install features such as Georgian-style windows in a new property to give it a period feel, but only a building that was actually constructed during the Georgian period will be authentic. Older properties often have other desirable features such as high, decorated ceilings (although rooms with high ceilings can cost more to heat), original fireplaces and attractive coloured glasswork built into the windows.

Try as one might, it is very difficult to make a new property feel like a characterful older one simply by adding period-style decoration and furniture. The general proportions and uniformity of room shape in many new properties just do not allow it to work. Victorian furniture will always look best in a real Victorian house, for example. After all, the furniture maker had just this sort of abode in mind when the furniture was made. An old property is also likely to be in a well-established road or district of similar-aged, distinctive buildings.

A garden

Whether you buy a new house or an old one, the chances are that it will have a garden. As we have seen, this can be a boon if you have children or pets. Depending on its size, you can use it for informal entertaining and to give vent to your horticultural skills. You may even decide to turn part of it over for vegetables, helping to keep down the cost of living while providing you with a supply of fresh seasonal food. Although a garden does not necessarily cost much to tend, apart from the purchase of some tools, it can prove extremely time-consuming to keep even a modest-sized one looking really neat and tidy – an important consideration if you like to spend the warmer months of the year doing something else.

Viewing

Properties for sale are advertised in many of the same outlets as rented properties. Although properties for sale do not usually go as quickly as rented ones, it pays to move fast if you find your absolute dream abode – the chances are that there will be others who are thinking likewise.

When you see a property you like, it is customary to make an appointment to view it. This is usually arranged through the estate agents who are handling the sale for the seller (also known as the vendor), but may be directly with the seller. (Check the advertisement or the 'For Sale' board outside the property.) Looking over a property should be a carefully considered task, and it can sometimes be great fun as well. Here are some tips on finding your ideal home.

First of all, look at the surrounding area. If the property is on a main road, is this going to be a problem, because of noise, or a danger for your children or pets? Visit the location during the rush hour to get a sense of the traffic conditions at their worst; a visit later in the day may give a false impression of tranquillity. Is there a school very close by? This could be noisy at certain times of the day and you could have a stream of traffic doing the twice-daily 'school run'. If you prefer a quiet life, is there a communal play area very close to your property that could be noisy? Is the property close to a flight path or a railway line? If so, how often do aeroplanes and trains pass by? How is the property served for local schools, shops and other amenities? Overall, how do the nearby streets and houses look – in other words, what is the general neighbourhood like? Is this an established neighbourhood, an up-and-coming one or a deteriorating neighbourhood? Do adjoining properties appear to be in good condition from the outside? Have the neighbours got rusty, half-dismantled cars or other eyesores in their front drive? Has a neighbour got a caravan parked so that it is blocking your view or obstructing the natural light into your property?

The aspect of the property (the direction it faces) is important. The natural light that a property receives can make a big difference to its general ambience – and indeed, to the quality of living inside. Some buildings have rooms that get sunlight in the morning, and others do not get lit until the afternoon's rays strike them. A few buildings seem to get almost no direct sunlight at all. If the property has a garden, it is generally preferable if the garden faces south. By noting which way the building faces and where the sun rises in the morning and sets in the afternoon, you can easily work out what sort of light the property will get.

Look at the general state of repair as seen from the outside. Check the condition of window frames, soffits and fascias. Are they low-maintenance UPVC or plastic? If so, have they been faded by the sun's ultraviolet rays? Do the doors and other woodwork need repainting? Look at the garden – is it well kept? (This is often an indication as to the general attitude of the owner to maintenance of the whole property.) Has the property got any features you do not like and that may be difficult or expensive to change? Are there any missing tiles on the roof or any cracked windows? If the property is a flat or a maisonette, check the condition of any communal walkways and stairs. If there is a lift, see if it is working. If there is a shared garden or outside area, check your access to it.

Overall, try to analyse your general feeling about the property as you walk up to the front door. Could you see yourself happily living here? If so, let's go inside!

The impression you get when walking through the door of a property for the first time will often have an enormous influence on whether or not you ultimately like the place. Because of this, people sometimes ensure fresh coffee is brewing or bread is in the oven when potential buyers come to view, because these aromas help to add a homely ambience. However, try not to let these superficial impressions colour your overall opinion of the place. When you view a property, the owner (or the owner's agent) will probably show you round room by room. Take your time over this and have a really good look. Are you satisfied that all the rooms are functional in terms of their size, shape and their location within the property? Try to imagine each room without any furniture. This will help you to envisage the way it will look before you add your own belongings. If there are particular things that you really want from a home – perhaps an open fire – make sure these features are present or at least achievable. Listen carefully to what the seller is telling you about the property in general and about specific details such as any improvements they have made, where power points are located and so on. Don't be afraid to ask questions, and to take measurements and other notes if you wish. After all, the seller wants someone to buy the property and should be only too pleased to encourage interest provided they consider you to be genuine. Ask what is included in the sale by way of fixtures and fittings (these usually refer to items such as wall lights, but do not assume these are automatically included).

Look carefully to see if there are any obvious faults such as damp patches or sagging floorboards. It is also worth noting the condition of the decoration. Do you like the décor, or will the property need a complete and costly makeover? How modern are the bathroom and kitchen fittings? What is the view like from all of the windows? Enquire about the quality of the television and radio signals; some properties, and even whole areas, get poor reception due to the proximity of tall trees and other buildings close by, or because the property is situated in a dip or is on the edge of the transmission range. Does your mobile phone work?

Always take with you the property details supplied by the estate agent if you have them. They may help to remind you about some aspect of the property that you want to investigate. It should be remembered, however, that what is described on the estate agent's property details is not legally binding, although action against the agent may be possible if particulars are incorrect or misleading.

If there is a garden, go outside and walk round that too. Do you like the way it is laid out? Is it a garden you could manage? If not, could it be easily changed to suit you? Are you overlooked by neighbours? Are there any visible eyesores (such as a neighbour's rubbish)? If you have young children, has it got a pond or any other features that might be dangerous? Is there road or other noise that might spoil your enjoyment of the garden? Does the garden have tall trees that shade the light from the garden, and if so, is there any sort of preservation order preventing them from being cut back?

More questions to ask

Once you have been round the house, ask the vendor anything else that you want to know. Why are they selling the house? What are the neighbours like? Can you hear them through the walls? The seller may not want to tell you things that might jeopardise a sale, but you can at least ask! Most of us think of other questions we should have asked once we have left the property. Don't be afraid to call the seller or the agent to ask more questions if something else occurs to you. It is also quite usual to ask to make a second visit – indeed, this is recommended.

These tips may help you avoid some of the pitfalls when buying a property – and of course, many of them are also useful when it comes to looking for somewhere to rent. After all, you always want to live somewhere pleasant. Taking careful note of any genuine shortcomings as you go round can help you strike a better deal when it comes to agreeing a price. However, be sure that what you point out are real defects; no seller is going to reduce the price just because you don't like the decoration and will want to change it all.

If you decide that you wish to buy the house, it is usual to make an offer. You can do this through the estate agent or direct to the seller. Houses and flats seldom sell for exactly the price they are advertised, unless they are new. It isn't sensible to offer a ridiculously low price, but if you can judge that the seller is anxious to sell quickly, or if extensive repairs are required, you may be able to negotiate a lower price, and get a real bargain. You may have also looked at similar properties in the area and know that the asking price for this property is too high. If you have no property of your own to sell, and you have already arranged finance, such as a mortgage (see page 60), to cover the asking price, this also puts you in a strong bargaining position.

Remember, however, that many house sales are part of a 'chain', in which each buyer is also trying to sell their own property and so on, so there may still be a time delay before you can move in. It is not unknown for a sale to collapse altogether because the chain has broken (in other words, because someone in the chain cannot sell their house or a house has been withdrawn from sale). Do be prepared for last-minute disappointment.

Mortgages

Once you have found your ideal property, you have to get together the money to buy it. Most properties are purchased with the aid of a mortgage. This is essentially a loan, given against the value of the property you wish to buy. If you default on your payments for any reason, the lender (the company providing the loan) can recover their losses by repossessing the property and selling it.

You can arrange to have a mortgage in your joint names. There are advantages and disadvantages on both sides, and you will have to discuss this with your partner. For example, if the mortgage is in only one partner's name, then the other partner is not, effectively, an owner of the property. They will not be able to benefit from the increase in the property's value if it is sold, following a break-up, nor would they become the owner if their partner dies (as would be the case for a married couple). In addition, although there are ways that a partner can avoid eviction following a break-up, it is clearly going to be harder if the property is owned by the other party. On the plus side, the partner who does not own the property will not be responsible for mortgage payments under any circumstances, which will make things simpler if there is a break-up.

On the whole, I would recommend that you have your mortgage in joint names. Many lenders will insist on it for a variety of reasons, and they will probably also insist that the property is also owned in joint names. Both of these will make things easier for a surviving partner in the event of the death of the other. If there is a default by one of the two partners paying the mortgage, or one dies, the mortgage lender may allow the other partner to continue with the mortgage alone, depending on the level of their income, of course. You would have to discuss this with your lender. It is also important to have a will that ensures the interest of the surviving partner in the property if one partner dies.

You should be aware that a lender may not grant a joint mortgage – or any mortgage at all – if one partner has a bad credit record, even if the other has a perfectly blameless record.

There are several ways of obtaining a mortgage. Building societies and banks are among the most common sources but there are also other companies dedicated to providing loans. The repayment rates tend to vary according to the level of interest rates, and they also vary from lender to lender, so you must be prepared to shop around to see what looks competitive at the time. It is also important to establish the

Annual Percentage Rate (usually known as the APR) in order to ascertain the total amount of interest payable over the life of the loan.

Not only do rates vary, but so does the type of mortgage available. Repayment mortgages and endowment mortgages are the most common, although the latter are less in favour now than previously. Other types include pension-linked and interest-only mortgages. Personal equity plans (PEPs) and individual share accounts (ISAs) offer further options for the repayment of mortgage accounts. Your lender will explain the differences, and the advantages of the different schemes, to help you decide which is best for you. Remember, however, that many banks and building societies also offer a whole range of other financial services such as pensions and insurance as part of their portfolio. Try to make it clear to your lender the type of scheme you have in mind, so that they can offer the most appropriate type of mortgage, tailored to your needs and circumstances.

It pays to compare schemes between several lenders, even if they seem superficially the same. Some may impose penalties for paying the mortgage early, for instance, or may insist on a particular policy being used to insure the building. This may turn out to be a less competitive policy than one you might be able to source yourself. It is also possible to seek the advice of an independent financial adviser to establish which lenders and types of loan are most competitive and most suitable for your circumstances.

When you have decided what sort of loan you want and where you want to get it from, you will inevitably be required to fill in forms regarding your personal and financial details. The forms may ask whether you have ever been refused a loan or been served with a court judgment. Your answers will then be used to assess your suitability for a loan and to satisfy the lender that you can afford to repay the loan. It is important to be truthful when answering these questions, since knowingly giving false information could be an offence. Your lender will do their best to provide a loan, and you can always discuss any issues that arise as a result of the answers you give.

Before a loan is granted on a property, the lender will carry out a detailed structural inspection of the property known as a survey. This will assess its general condition to ensure it is worth the money they are loaning you to buy it. Occasionally, the survey will highlight problems, such as subsidence or rot, that must be attended to either before a loan is granted or as part of the loan agreement. The surveyor may come to the conclusion that the property only warrants a smaller loan than the one you are seeking. In this instance you may need to renegotiate the price with the seller or seek additional funds elsewhere. Beware, however, that if more than one loan is sought on a property, the consent of the first mortgagee is required before obtaining the second mortgage.

Conveyancing

Once your offer on a house has been accepted by the seller and you have your loan offer from the bank or building society, the work of conveyancing must start. Some people take care of this themselves – and there are self-help packs and even books that show you how to do this – but most home-buyers prefer to leave it to solicitors who are trained to carry out the work.

Conveyancing involves not only drawing up the legal documents for the sale and purchase of the property but also obtaining local and land registry searches, checks on the legal title to the land and land registration. Local land searches are designed to identify any proposed roads, planned buildings or other matters that may be detrimental to the value of the property, for example. Some of these proposals, if carried out, may also effect the quality of life you enjoy in your home, and so they should be taken seriously and investigated. These searches should also highlight public rights of way and other matters that may not be obvious at first sight. For example, a search may reveal that there is a public right of way across your property. There have even been extreme cases where it was discovered that a right of way actually existed through the property itself! Land registration lists you as the owner(s) of the property and indicates exactly the boundaries of your land.

As I said earlier, buying a house is a big undertaking. Your conveyancing solicitor should go through the details of the sale contract with you, and your borrower should explain the terms of the mortgage offer. However, once you have signed everything, you are legally bound by the terms of the agreements. There may be clauses, known as covenants, that restrict what you can do to the property and these may, for example, restrict you from undertaking structural changes. This is particularly the case if your property is part of a recent housing development or if there is a preservation order on the property due to its historical importance. In some owner–occupier properties – this is usually more common in blocks of private flats – it may not be permitted for you to keep pets such as cats or dogs. It is worth stating again here that if you default or fall behind on the payments of your mortgage, the lender could repossess the property and evict you.

Other costs

In addition to everything described in the previous section, there are other costs directly associated with the legalities of buying a property, which must be budgeted for. These include solicitors' fees for the work described above, the costs of searches, land registry fees and stamp duty. These costs will all be documented when the purchase agreement for the property is drawn up by your solicitor.

You may need to pay for a removal firm to transport your furniture from a previous address. It is usual to ask two or three removal firms to give you a price (known as a quotation) for this work, since prices can vary quite widely. Many couples setting up home together for the first time usually find it easier and less expensive to do the job themselves using a hired van, however.

You may also need to pay for the professional installation of equipment such as washing machines, telephone points, television aerials, satellite dishes and so on.

From the first day that you take possession of your new home, you will be required to start paying for the supply of services such as water. As a property owner, you will also have to pay a community charge. This is your contribution for services such as refuse collection, upkeep of the local roads and footpaths, policing and streetlighting.

Buying your own home also means that you will need to have your own furniture, kitchen equipment and all the items that are usually already provided in furnished accommodation. It may be that you own many of these already, of course – from previous relationships or from your previous accommodation – and they can help to reduce your initial outgoings considerably. The chapter entitled Furnishing and Running Your Home lists the most important items you will need to help you plan for this.

7

furnishing and running your home

A home is in many ways a reflection of what you put into it, and it is only natural that any couple living together will want to make their own place unique, homely and special. However, don't be in too great a rush to spend money on things for your home. You may find that your requirements and priorities change quickly once you have settled in and taken stock.

What have we got?

In the light of what I've just said, instead of starting to think about what you need, it is perhaps a better idea first of all to establish exactly what you have already got. It's a good idea to draw up a list.

If you and your partner have previously lived away from home or have divided up the contents of previous homes with former partners, the chances are that you own a fairly substantial amount of household goods already, including furniture, ornaments and kitchenware. Add all of these to your list.

If you are moving into furnished rented accommodation, many necessary household items will already be there. They may be fairly cheap and cheerful examples, however, so you might still want to buy your own – but put them on the list for the time being.

If you are buying your home, you may find that certain items, such as curtains, carpets and light fittings, are included as part of the sale. You may also be able to come to an arrangement over the purchase of other items. If there is anything that interests you and that you need, ask the vendor whether they would be prepared to sell it. If you are embarrassed to ask for specific items, simply enquire if anything else is included in the sale. Someone moving into a smaller property, or one that has different décor, may have no use for even large items of furniture and may have been planning to sell certain things anyway.

Incidentally, if there are any removable features that particularly attract you to a property – perhaps a fire surround or an unusual door-knocker – be sure to get confirmation that they are included in the sale, too. If not, try to negotiate a price.

What do we want to keep?

Once you have listed everything you both own, you may find you have more than you need, so you must decide what you are going to do with the extra items. It is not a good idea to get rid of everything just because, for example, you are moving into rented accommodation and you don't have space for it. If your aim is to buy your own property in due course, then it is worth keeping things that you like. Large items can be put into storage – look in your Yellow Pages for a specialist firm – but this is an expensive option, so use it with care and remember to balance the cost of storage against the replacement cost if you simply get rid of the item now. It may be possible to lodge smaller pieces with friends or relatives.

The first course of action is to look at the list and see how much duplication there is. If you have both lived in your own homes, you will almost certainly find that you have a surplus toaster and kettle, not to mention numerous kitchen utensils, a television and perhaps even large items of furniture. Any duplicated items you don't need when setting up together are really only clutter, so select the best example and get rid of the other one. The rejects may only really be fit for the bin anyway, but reasonable items can always find a new home through the small ads or in car boot sales. If you don't want to advertise anything, charity shops, scout groups and other organisations may also be grateful for any unwanted items that they can resell.

It sounds so simple in theory, but in practice, whose duplicated item you get rid of, and whose you keep, can be a rich source of argument. To make the choice simpler, try to agree together some sort of vision of how you both want your home to look. At the same time, this is a good opportunity to draw up a list of which items you jointly own and which are owned individually. This can be invaluable to avoid acrimony should you break up at some point in the future. (If you prefer not to think in such pessimistic terms, remember that it will also stop your partner from throwing out some prized possession of yours, which they loathe, on the grounds that they thought it was theirs.)

There will probably be plenty of things that you think are indispensable but which your partner does not. Those old cushions dating back from your student days may have some sentimental memories for you, but if they are, in reality, tasteless and dated, your partner is unlikely to want to give them house room – and neither should you.

Conversely, if there are items that you don't want to use now – even though you can – it is extremely unlikely that you will want to use them in the future. You should probably consider getting rid of them before you move in.

Some duplicated items are definitely worth keeping, however. These include good sets of drinking glasses, crockery and cutlery, rugs, good bed linen and attractive pictures and prints. In other words, things that break, things you never seem to have enough of and items that can quickly make a new home attractive and welcoming. If you have more than one television or sound system between you, again, keep them both if possible. A spare is useful, and two televisions stop a lot of arguments about which programmes to watch!

Essentials

If you are starting from scratch, you need to draw up a list of the items that you consider absolutely essential. I have put together a suggested list – although some, admittedly, are more essential than others.

Once you have drawn up your list, shop around. Stores and other retail outlets compete avidly for your business, so look for deals such as interest-free credit, and delayed payment terms that offer incentives like 'Nothing to pay for two years'. Of course, you do not have to buy everything new. Almost anything you want can be obtained second-hand through classified advertisements, shop window advertisements, bric-a-brac shops, car boot sales and other outlets. It is astonishingly easy to pick up really good-quality things at bargain prices – perhaps this is an indication of how frequently people move nowadays from one home and relationship to another.

Furniture

Beds and sofas: First priority for most people is the bed. Buy a good-quality one if possible. At least buy the best you can afford, even if it means doing without something else for a while. A good bed will last longer and should give you a better night's sleep. Beds come in a range of widths. The most common width for a double bed is 4ft 6in, but 5ft and even 6ft beds are now quite common. Many beds have separate drawers built into the base. These are extremely useful for storage if space is tight.

You must both go to choose your bed – you need to test it by lying on it together (seriously!) and you should try out several before you decide. Make sure that it is long enough – built-in footboards can be a problem for tall people who like to stretch full length in bed. This may not be apparent in the store, because when you test the bed on the shop floor you will probably lie with your head higher up the bed than is the case when you are sleeping in bed using pillows. Try to use your imagination and really snuggle down! Make sure you try lying on your side as well as on your back – women in particular may find it difficult to get comfortable on their side if a mattress is too firm. Check that the bed you choose has universal fittings for a headboard so that you can attach one of your choice if you wish.

Sofa beds are an excellent idea, especially if space and funds are short. But beware, while some are very comfortable, others will make you feel you'd rather sleep in a chair and it does seem to be a case of 'you get what you pay for'. Buy the best you can afford. By the way, even if you have a bed already, don't turn down an offer of a sofa bed if one comes your way. These, and folding guest beds, are invaluable for putting up friends and visiting children.

A sofa is an expensive item and, as with beds, you should try out several before you buy. Again, you get what you pay for, so don't be fooled by something cheap that looks good in the showroom: poor-quality cushions and backrests can sag very quickly with use. Remember that you may want to co-ordinate your furniture with carpets and other soft furnishings in due course, so don't choose a wild pattern that looks great on its own but matches nothing. If you buy a sofa in a light-coloured fabric, make sure that it can be removed for easy cleaning (preferably washing) or put a throw over it for everyday use to keep it looking good.

Tables and chairs: Plenty of people eat almost all of their meals by balancing their plates on their laps, but this may be a skill that you don't want to learn, so you will need a table and chairs. Apart from anything, it is rather anti-social to invite guests round for a meal and not have anywhere suitable for them to eat. Remember that tables are amongst the easiest items of furniture to dress up, so if you have an old one that can be revived with a coat of paint or covered with a tablecloth, forget buying and make do. If you must buy and space is at a premium, folding, extending and gateleg tables are all ideal for saving space and will provide you with the option to accommodate more people when you need to. Paint chairs to match. If you like the look of wooden rather than upholstered seats, buy a few cushions to throw on them if you or your friends are going to be sitting on them for any length of time.

Storage: Good storage is essential if you are to keep your home tidy but this does not have to be expensive. Clothes can be inexpensively and neatly stored on clothes racks (often known as tidy rails) or in lightweight covered wardrobes, and there are dozens of kinds of cheap, simple storage systems for smaller items. Look out for wire or wicker baskets and open shelving. Browse some furniture catalogues or look around a few department stores for ideas and make a list of what you need. Remember again that many useful items can be purchased second-hand.

Television and stereo: Most people would not dream of doing without a television and stereo music system. These are arguably not essential items, but TV and radio are informative as well as entertaining and if you're strapped for cash, it's cheaper to stay in than go out. If you look like having arguments over what to watch on television, you may want to have a smaller set in the bedroom. You may need to discuss – and agree on – whether you want to have the additional expense of satellite or cable television. If you do, remember to take it into consideration when deciding who pays for what (see page 30).

Linen and soft furnishings

Bedlinen: Some people prefer sheets and blankets on their bed, and others prefer to use a duvet. It's purely a matter of choice, although it's quicker to make a bed with a duvet on it. The thermal insulation of a duvet is measured by its tog rating. This should be indicated clearly on the duvet when you buy it. The higher the tog number, the warmer the duvet. The one big drawback is that duvets don't offer the flexibility of blankets, which you can add or remove as the temperature falls and rises, so you may need a winter duvet as well as a summer one. If you choose a duvet, you also need to buy washable duvet covers. Pillows come with a wide variety of fillings, either synthetic or feather. Synthetic fillings are washable and are more suitable for people who suffer from allergies, so if your partner is asthmatic, don't be surprised if they refuse to sleep on your best luxury duck-down pillows. Pillows will require separate, washable pillow cases.

Towels: You can get by with just a few towels to begin with, although you will need replacements when one set is being washed. Hand towels and bath towels are both essential. Good-quality cotton towels cost more but last longer and dry you better. Don't forget that you may also need guest towels; it isn't really acceptable for guests to be expected to use towels that you are using at the same time.

Curtains and cushions: If you think that curtains are a waste of money, think again. Not only do curtains provide privacy, but they also keep fuel bills down by reducing heat loss from windows and doors. You can buy ready-made curtains to fit many sizes of windows but the latest tab-top styles, which hang on a pole, are simple to make. If you want something more elaborate, go to a department store to look at the range of curtain fittings and rails.

A few bright cushions are a good buy – they will make even the bleakest rented flat look cosy in minutes.

Kitchen equipment

Cooker: Your choice of a gas or an electric cooker may be limited by what utility is supplied to the property. There is a bewildering range of both types, but don't get carried away and buy a double oven with six burners on the hob and a special griddle plate unless you are a really dedicated cook.

Contrary to what many people seem to think nowadays, a microwave cooker is not essential, but it is particularly useful for busy people and can be a quick and economical way of preparing some meals.

Fridge: You really can't do without a fridge but fortunately they are not expensive. Don't buy a massive one if there are just the two of you – one that fits under the worktop will be perfectly adequate. You don't actually need a freezer, but if you have the money, a popular option is to buy a combined fridge-freezer. Usually the top half of the unit comprises the fridge, and the bottom half the freezer. Apart from the sheer convenience, a freezer allows you to save money by cooking and freezing food in bulk and enables you to take advantage of special offers and other foodstore bargains. The icebox in a fridge is no substitute – it will keep food icy cold for a while but it won't allow you to keep frozen food for months like a proper freezer will.

Washing machine/dryer: You can do without a washing machine if you can get to a laundrette – and not so long ago, most people did – but it's much easier to have your own. Even if you do some washing by hand, you can spin the clothes in the machine and they'll dry much quicker. You may also want to buy a tumble-dryer if you have room – particularly if you have no facilities for drying washing outside. There are combination washer/dryers on the market, which save space, but they are expensive to buy and run. You will certainly need an ironing board and iron.

Vacuum cleaner: Unless your home has only hard floor surfaces, such as wood block and tiles, a vacuum cleaner is an essential. There are many types to choose from – upright models, cylinder models and multifunction cleaners that shampoo carpets as well as vacuum up dirt. It's a matter of choice and budget.

Kitchen utensils

Cooking utensils: You will need mixing bowls, spoons, pans, saucepans, spatulas, kitchen knives, egg cups, waste bin, salt, pepper and spice dispensers, table mats, storage jars and possibly even scales – the list just goes on and on. Fortunately, this is where most of us can bring something into a partnership – we all seem to have some kitchen items even if it's just a corkscrew and a chopping board. Check your list of what you've got (see page 65) and browse through a kitchenware catalogue before you buy; this will help you choose the most needed items first.

Crockery, glasses and cutlery: They're not strictly utensils, but crockery, drinking glasses and cutlery will be needed, too. Once again, check your list and when you set out to buy, remember that there may not always be just the two of you eating so buy sets of at least four, more if you can afford it. You will need dinner plates, side plates, bowls (choose a design that will do for both soup and desserts), cups and saucers. To this, you can add other matching items such as gravy boat, milk jug, sugar bowl and tea and coffee pots if you wish.

You will need lots of drinking glasses, so keep all you have. (This may not apply if one of you has a collection with particularly tasteless pictures etched on them, of course.) If you have lots of odd ones, keep them for everyday use – you'll soon smash your way through them. If you are buying new glasses, choose a design and stick to it. As a minimum, you will probably want wine glasses, short tumblers for spirits and taller glasses for long drinks and beers.

When buying cutlery, you will get the best value if you buy a canteen, containing at least six sets of full place settings. Styles vary from the very formal and ornate to the most contemporary and plain. If you can't manage this, many kitchen shops sell knives, forks and spoons individually in a variety of styles – remember to buy lots of teaspoons. Somehow there are never enough. Whatever you buy, make sure they are dishwasher-proof. Even if you haven't got a dishwasher now, you may buy one in the future.

Miscellaneous

There are many other items that you will probably need sooner or later, including occasional lamps and tables, rugs and mirrors. These are not essential and you can buy them as you go along.

If you have a garden, you will need a few basic tools to keep it looking neat and tidy or it will quickly turn into a jungle. Any area of lawn will require regular cutting. A very tiny lawn can be cut with garden shears, but proper lawn mowers are the ideal tool. Buy one in a size and style to suit your needs and your pocket. You will also find the following useful: garden spade, fork, rake, garden broom, watering can, gardening gloves and trowel. You may also need a wheelbarrow. In time you can buy other items for tackling more specialised jobs.

DIY

Sooner or later you will want to put up a mirror, a shelf or a picture and you may also find you have to put together furniture that comes in a flatpack for home assembly. Having the correct tools for the job makes any task quicker and simpler. Tools are readily available through hardware stores and other outlets, and car boot sales are another good source. If you are a DIY novice, start with a few tools to enable you to do simple tasks.

Basic tool kit

Here is a list of the most useful and versatile tools for tackling domestic jobs like the ones described above, as well as many other tasks in the home and garden. You don't have to buy them all at once – just when the need arises.

Screwdrivers: Buy at least one medium-sized screwdriver for general work and a small one for replacing fuses and changing plugs. Many self-assembly units are fixed together using cross-slotted screws, so you will also need Phillips screwdrivers, which are designed for these.

Hammer: A medium-weight hammer incorporating a 'claw' for removing old nails is ideal. Look for those with rubber handles for improving grip and absorbing the shock of impact.

Spirit level: An essential item for ensuring shelves, pictures and so on are level.

Pliers: A general-purpose pair of pliers will usually incorporate a useful wire-cutting tool. Long-nosed pliers are more useful for intricate work.

Saw: For general carpentry (for example, cutting wood for shelves) a 20in panel saw is ideal. A hacksaw for cutting metal is also very useful when cutting tubing (such as wardrobe rails) and other general metalwork.

Drill: A hand drill is useful for making holes in wood or metal, but if you intend to drill into walls or masonry, then an electric drill is really a must. Cordless electric drills, which are powered by their own rechargeable batteries, are particularly easy to handle in awkward places, but are not always as powerful as their mains-driven counterparts. Some drills have a hammer-drill function that allows the drill to penetrate masonry more easily.

You will need several drill bits – these are the actual drilling tools that fit into the front of the drill (the chuck). Drill bits can be purchased separately, but it is possible to buy them in a pack of varying sizes and designs for drilling into different materials, such as wood, metal or masonry. Most drills can also be adapted for screwing, sanding, cutting and performing other tasks, simply by fitting different tools to the drill's chuck.

Useful extras

A steel tape measure is useful. Buy screws, nails and wallplugs as you need them – you can buy 'variety' packs but they often fail to contain the exact size you want! A pipe detector (see page 74) is an invaluable tool for detecting electrical wiring, water pipes and other metal objects within walls. Cutting or drilling 'blind' into such structures could prove highly expensive – and dangerous.

Decorating

A few extra tools will be required if you are going to give your new home a fresh look! First, you may need a small palette knife to apply filler to cracks in walls and woodwork, and sandpaper of different grades for smoothing surfaces before you paint. You will also need a selection of paint brushes. For wallpapering, the most important tools are a scraper (for removing old paper), a paste brush, a wallpaper brush (for smoothing out the wallpaper when it is on the wall) and a seam roller (for ensuring the edges of the wallpaper lie flat). A plumb line is also needed for ensuring the edge of the wallpaper is exactly vertical before you paste it up. You can buy one, but it is a simple task to make your own, using a small weight (such as a small nut or bolt) tied to a long piece of thin cord.

Home improvement and safety

Decorating and other home DIY, as well as gardening, should be relaxing, safe and rewarding pastimes. Every year, however, thousands of people are injured at home – and some are even killed – while they attempt to carry out home improvements. Pipe detectors, which I mentioned above, are sold in DIY stores and hardware stores, and can prevent accidents caused by drilling or nailing through hidden pipes or electric cables – they emit an audible signal when drawn across an area of wall, ceiling or floor that may be concealing such structures.

Another extremely useful and inexpensive piece of equipment is an RCD adaptor. This simply plugs into your mains electrical socket, and you then put the plug from your appliance into the adaptor. The adaptor monitors electricity flow and switches off the power to the appliance immediately it senses a variation, providing life-saving protection should you accidentally damage a cable. It should be used with all power tools, especially electrically driven garden tools and mowers.

Still on the subject of safety, it is a very good idea to fit smoke alarms or detectors to help protect you in the case of fire in your home. These are simple devices to install, and it is best to fit one on each level of your home or as recommended by the suppliers of the appliance. You could also consider buying a small fire extinguisher and/or a fire blanket – many people keep one in the kitchen.

Protecting your home and belongings

There is much you can do to minimise the risk of being burgled, and many of the steps you can take apply to tenants in rented property as well as to homeowners. Most thieves are so-called 'opportunists' – they are looking for somewhere that is easy and quick to break into and in which it is easy to find items to steal. Therefore the first task is to make your property less attractive to a would-be thief.

Fit window locks. They aren't expensive, and if you cannot fit them yourself, a handyman will do the job for you at a reasonable price. Professionally fitted double-glazed windows are usually more secure than ordinary ones and often have locks already fitted.

Fit good locks on all outside doors. Those fitted as standard, particularly yale locks, are often woefully inadequate – a 5-lever mortise lock is the minimum that should be fitted. Although front doors are often fairly secure, it is the back or side doors that are more attractive to a thief. Reinforce door panels if they are simply made of plywood by adding extra thick wood panels on the inside, or by fitting a mesh guard. This can be painted to match the door and is almost invisible. For extra security, fit bolts that lock the door into the door frame.

A further deterrent is a burglar alarm. There are some devices that you can fit yourself, and others that require professional installation. Most have an alarm box, which is fitted in a prominent position high up on one of the walls of the property, to act as a visible warning to would-be thieves.

More and more property owners are fitting security lights. Security lights usually incorporate a sensor that switches on a powerful light beam when it detects movement. An adjustable timer controls the length of time the light stays on. They are designed to work in low light levels only, so that they do not come on unnecessarily during the day.

It almost goes without saying that you should keep valuables such as jewellery, car keys and so on in a secure place. It is also advisable not to keep excessive amounts of cash in your home – put it into an account where it can earn interest. If you want to keep valuables at home, one way of helping to reduce the loss is by fitting a safe. A small, strong safe can be bolted securely to a wall inside a cupboard.

With the exception of the alarm system, none of the above is very expensive. You may also find that your insurance company will reduce your premiums if you have security devices fitted, thus saving you money as well as giving you peace of mind.

Making your home economical to run

There are lots of DIY jobs you can do to keep your bills down. First, if your property has wood-framed windows and external wooden trim, it pays to keep them painted regularly. You may find it necessary to repaint parts of the external woodwork every couple of years or so to avoid the need to replace rotted window frames or other parts.

Next, you can reduce your heating bills by ensuring your valuable heat does not escape too fast. Most houses and flats have some form of loft insulation – usually glass fibre wool or foam crumbs – to help keep heating bills lower and save energy. However, many properties have only a minimal amount of insulation. If your property has less than 6 in (15 cm) of insulation, you should add some more. It is quite easy to do this yourself. Insulation comes in rolls (or in bags in the case of crumbs) which you simply spread between the joists in the loft, over entry hatches and anywhere else from which heat may escape. Wear gloves and a face mask when rolling out glass fibre wool, since it can irritate your skin and lungs.

Improve the heat retention in the rest of the property. Draught excluders, which are self-adhesive or are tacked with small nails to the door and window frames, can prevent heat loss. A more effective solution is to fit double glazing. You can buy an inexpensive version of this which simply fits inside the window frame or window recess, but it is only partially effective because the air trapped between the original glass and the additional panes is usually not perfectly still, and this reduces the efficiency of the system. The best results, however, if you can afford it, will come from a specially manufactured system of double glazing for windows and doors, fitted by experts.

Another useful form of heat retention is cavity wall insulation, but this is another job for the professionals.

One important point to remember with all these methods of insulation is that although these remedies are effective in reducing heat loss, they can be expensive to install. Although you may feel the benefits immediately in terms of cosier surroundings, it will take some time for you to get your money back through reduced bills. If you are likely to be moving house within a few years, such measures may therefore not be fully cost-effective – although they will undoubtedly add to the desirability of your property if you ever decide to put it on the market again.

Other easy ways to save money about the house

- Make sure your hot water tank (usually situated in the airing cupboard) is lagged to help retain heat. Lagging jackets can be purchased at DIY stores, but at a pinch you could simply wrap the tank in old blankets or similar materials.
- Change washers on leaking or dripping taps.
- Use energy-saving bulbs.
- Fit thermostats to radiators.
- Set up a washing line so you don't need to use a tumble-dryer if the weather is fine.

8

children

For many couples who live together, children will already be, or may become, an important part of the relationship jigsaw. Whether it be marriage or cohabitation, the presence of children fundamentally changes the status quo in a multitude of different ways, usually for ever. Children can, and normally do, affect every aspect of our lives – emotional, financial and legal. Equally, we, as parents, step-parents or just caring adults, have an effect on almost everything that is important in their lives, including their emotional well-being, their happiness and their ability to grow up to be decent human beings.

This book is not designed to try to provide a guide to good parenting – there is already a host of excellent books available on the subject (and in my opinion, your family, friends and your own instinctive judgment may be the best guides in such matters). What is intended here is a discussion of some of the ways that you can tackle the special problems and other issues that often arise when there are children involved in a living-together relationship, and to outline some of the legal differences compared with marriage. Note, however, that the law is not the same everywhere. There are variations within different parts of the UK, for example. Seek professional legal advice if you have any uncertainty about how the law affects you.

Children in a cohabiting relationship

Once upon a time, people got married and then had children. Nowadays, the situation is often very different. Many couples decide to live together first, then get married once the female partner discovers that she is pregnant. Though your great aunt may sniff at the order of events, there are no long-term complications: the child is born to a married couple.

79

You may decide alternatively that you, a cohabiting couple, would like to have children but do not intend to get married at any stage. This may feel like a non-decision to you, but it should not be undertaken lightly. You should, for example, be prepared for the law to view your situation differently from married couples in some fundamental ways (see below). You may also meet resistance and disapproval from other members of your own or your partner's family. For many people, the idea of children being born out of wedlock is upsetting to them and even nowadays it can have a social stigma. More importantly, in the longer term, it may even engender some resentment in the child, or a feeling of being somehow different. You and your partner must be prepared to have the confidence to deal with these problems.

Children and the law

Where children are concerned, there are considerable differences between the way the law regards married and unmarried couples. This applies right from the beginning, or perhaps more accurately, conception, for the male partner of a cohabiting couple, unlike his married counterpart, is not presumed to be the father of a child born to his partner. His name therefore cannot appear on the birth certificate without the presence and agreement of both the mother and the father, unless a court declares that he is the father. In the case of married couples, either parent can register the birth, giving the names of both the father and the mother.

The situation is much the same as regards responsibility for the children as they grow up. Under UK law, parental responsibility is defined as 'all the rights, duties, powers, responsibilities and authority which by law a parent of a child has in relation to the child and his property'. All parents, it is to be hoped, wish to bear some responsibility for the welfare and behaviour of their children, and by law married parents share this responsibility, which continues until the children are 18. They are also both responsible for supporting the children financially, even if the name of the father does not appear on the child's birth certificate. If the parents separate or divorce, this remains the case. Sometimes one parent will be awarded care and control and the children will live with that one parent, but both parents still share all parental responsibility for them. However, it may surprise you to know that in the eyes of the law unmarried parents do not actually share any rights where their children are concerned, even if they live together. These belong to the mother alone – an unmarried father enjoys no automatic parental responsibility for his own child.

This remains the case unless the mother and father make a formal agreement to change the situation, or, as may be the case in some circumstances, a court finds in favour of the father and makes a court order to this end. If the mother dies, the father may gain responsibility by becoming the child's guardian – but again, this would have to be the subject of an application to the courts. If a cohabiting couple separate, the father of their children has no rights or responsibilities towards them at all.

In the same way, homosexual and lesbian partners have no automatic parental responsibility for any children born by or to their partner. It is possible for them to apply to the courts for a joint residence order with the children's mother if this is appropriate, however, and this does give them certain limited rights.

I should mention here that whilst in the UK, and most of the Western hemisphere, the mother enjoys all the rights and responsibilities, there may be variations according to the laws of differing countries and even within those countries. (Scottish law, for example, is different from the law in England and Wales, and in the US, laws vary from one state to another.) In some parts of the world mothers may have no rights at all. It is important, therefore, to seek legal advice in the country in which you live so that you are fully aware of the situation in relation to your children.

Children from previous relationships

For many people, the decision to live with someone is a step they take following the break-up of a marriage or a previous relationship. Often, one or both of the partners in this new arrangement will already have had one or more children with their former partner. It can be difficult at times to integrate these children – whether they be your own or your new partner's – successfully into your new situation, and it needs to be done with patience and understanding. In all dealings with children, it is vital that their feelings and needs are taken into account as much as possible. The breakdown of a relationship is hugely unsettling for children, and they require reassurance and the knowledge that there will still be contact between them and their parents, even if it is on a different level than previously.

However, before children can even become part of a new relationship, there are issues that must be tackled first. So before you even think of moving your children in with your new partner (or vice versa), you and your partner need to sit down and discuss some major questions. Ideally, such discussions should also involve your ex-partner, the other parent of the children, but this may not be possible.

- If the children are not yet independent, who are they going to live with?
- How will the children be provided for financially?
- What other arrangements need to be put in place to reduce disruption to their lives?

In dealing with these issues, many relationship counsellors and family lawyers often talk about parental responsibilities rather than parental rights, and it is important not to lose sight of the difference between these terms. If you try to think of what is best for the children rather than what you want for yourself, you'll be on the right lines. Similarly, it is usual these days to talk in terms of 'residence' and 'contact' instead of 'custody' and 'access' when dealing with how to care for children and their needs, the idea being that these words are less confrontational.

Who will they live with?

Determining which parent a child is going to live with is always a sensitive issue. The situation may be further complicated if the parents have never been married. However, whatever the circumstances, you should try to deal with it as amicably as possible to help prevent the child feeling that he or she is part of the reason you are splitting up as a family. If you cannot decide this between yourself and your former partner, then a mediator or a solicitor may be able to help reach an agreement out of court.

If a solution cannot be found by any of these means, one of you can apply to the courts for a residence order. The court will listen to the case from each parent and may ask for reports from welfare officers before making its decision. Usually, a very young child who has been in the care of its mother since birth will be ordered to remain living with the mother. The court is also very unlikely to split up brothers and sisters.

A court will consider the child's welfare first and foremost and will consider especially the following:

- The child's needs (emotional, physical and educational)
- Any possible changes in the child's circumstances
- Any risks or harm that the child may have suffered or could suffer
- The child's age, sex, background and any characteristics that the court feels are relevant
- The ability of each parent to meet the child's needs
- The wishes of the child (taking into account the age of the child and his or her understanding of the situation)

Who is going to pay?

By law, as I've already said, both parents are responsible for financially maintaining their child. This is the case even if they have no contact with the child and even if the birth was not planned. When parents live apart, it is likely that the parent who does not live with the child will be expected to provide financial assistance to the other parent for bringing up the child. This period of support usually extends until the time the child has ceased full-time education.

This financial arrangement is often known as child support maintenance. The amount of maintenance may be determined by a court. Alternatively, a court may issue a maintenance order confirming an amount already agreed between both parents. A parent who defaults on these payments may be contacted by bodies such as the Child Support Agency, who will make efforts to ensure the payments are resumed. They have powers, for example, to arrange for part of the defaulting parent's wages to be deducted at source and paid directly to the Agency, who will then pass it on. Clearly, it is not in the interests of the child for there to be a break in the continuity of support.

When couples split up, there may also be the former home to consider. Sometimes one partner remains in the home but may be required to provide funds for the other partner to purchase new accommodation. Possibly the former home will be sold, and both partners will receive a share of the proceeds to finance new accommodation. Whatever route you take, expect to be worse off financially afterwards and possibly for some time to come.

Introducing them into your new relationship

The problems arising from your separation from your children's other parent will seem endless. But eventually, sooner or later, the questions of residency, contact and financial support will all be resolved. By then, it is possible that your children will have already met and know your new partner. Now you must all begin the process of continuing with your lives. This is rarely straightforward, and you as adults have by far the most to do to ensure it is a success.

Depending on the situation, several different 'relationship landscapes' are possible. There may be children living with you more or less permanently; the children may be yours alone, your partner's alone or they may belong to both you and your partner. There may be children from one partner's former relationship living more or less permanently in the home, and children from the other partner's relationship may be occasional visitors that stay from time to time. Or there may be no children living permanently in the home, but children from one or other partner's former relationship may be visitors. Within each of these landscapes there is a myriad of other factors that may affect everyone in the house: the personalities of each of the people involved, the ages of the children, the circumstances of the original break-up(s) and the circumstances of the new relationships.

It is clearly impossible here to provide a comprehensive guide on how to deal with each of these situations. Nevertheless, there are some basic ground rules to observe that can help in smoothing out what can often be a rocky road ahead. Some will obviously relate to you if you are the parent of the child, and others will be more pertinent if the child belongs to your new live-in partner.

If the child concerned is yours, do try if possible to maintain a reasonably amicable relationship with your child's other parent, even to the extent of continuing to celebrate events such as your child's birthday together. Bite your lip, grit your teeth and do anything you can to prevent having rows in front of the child. This will help to make your child feel more secure and will help him or her to realise that things may not be so bad after all. Having a good relationship with your ex-spouse or partner will also help to keep you 'in the loop' about things the children do at school and about their lives in general if you do not have regular contact. Sadly, many parents use their children as emotional weapons following a separation or a divorce. It is an all-too-common reaction for parents who feel injured to criticise and run down the other parent, sometimes turning the child against them. This does nothing to help the child, however, and no matter how tempted you may be, you should make every effort to curb such behaviour.

It is a good idea to work out, with your ex-partner if possible, a schedule of dates to cover visits and other contact times. Write them down and make sure you both have a copy. (You should try to ensure the dates go far enough ahead so that you can plan for holidays and so on. In particular, summer holidays and major events such as Christmas can be a source of tremendous aggravation.) Then, having made a list of dates, stick to it! You may have to move heaven and earth to keep to your original plans, but 'visiting' parents, especially, should try to maintain as much consistency as they possibly can and should ensure that their ex-partner does the same. Also, make sure you are both punctual in picking up, delivering or returning children after visits. And don't make plans that involve your children during their visits to the other parent.

The younger the children are at the time of the break-up, the easier it will normally be for them to come to terms with the situation. If they are old enough to understand what is going on, it will be necessary to handle things sensitively. Answer any questions they may ask. Make it clear that they were not in any way responsible for the break-up and that it doesn't mean they aren't loved just as much as before. Try to explain that although both parents will not always be at home together, there will still be plenty of contact and fun together. Also make it clear that you are still their mother or father and can still be there for them if there are problems.

Even if they are still living with you, you may need to find extra time for your children, at least initially, to help them over the absence of the other parent. If the child is not living with you, then time spent together will inevitably be more precious, and this can often bond together more closely parents and their children – who they may have taken for granted from time to time. This so-called 'quality time' does not need to be spent constantly doing something exciting. Trips to zoos and other amusements are great fun, but what the child really needs more than anything is your time and attention.

Often the most difficult relationship where children are concerned is the one between your new partner and your own children. Your children may resent this new person who they may regard as competing with them for your attention. If the separation from their mother or father was as a result of you meeting your new partner, then this may be a cause of resentment, too. They may react badly to anything that they perceive as your new partner acting as a surrogate parent.

Your partner may experience many of the same resentments. They may feel that your children are being difficult, surly, or even downright rude. It can often be worse when the children are only weekend or occasional visitors, because the bond or respect that begins to build often needs to be reforged on subsequent meetings. It can also be difficult for your partner to make any decisions about your children, however small and well-intended, and this can lead to a sense of detachment and isolation.

How well you all come to terms with this sometimes difficult situation depends to a large degree on the individuals concerned. But you and your partner, being the adults, will probably be expected to try hardest of all to make it work and to make the general atmosphere and environment as normal and happy as possible.

You will probably have to put just as much effort in if the children are not yours, but your partner's. First of all, there is the need to get to know each other and to gain mutual respect. Try to engage the children in conversation. Without bombarding them with too many questions, try to show you are taking an interest in them and what they are doing. Ask about their school, their pastimes and so on. Tell them something about yourself, too – what job you do, for instance. If they seem to show an interest, ask them to help you around the house or garden, but don't burden them with laborious tasks so that they become bored. If you do, they will probably give you a wide berth in future in case you ask them to do anything else of a similar nature! Be fulsome in your gratitude. If you have children of your own, you will probably know instinctively the kinds of things that children enjoy doing and this will make it easier in your relationship with them.

If your partner's children come to stay at weekends, try to make them feel as if this is their second home, rather than a place in which they are regarded as visitors. Otherwise, they will feel on edge and will find it harder to accept the situation. You should try to ensure that they don't feel unwilling to stay, because this will inevitably put a strain on your relationship with your partner. If you have space, make a permanent bedroom available for the children. Hard though it might be, try to avoid nagging them about untidiness and the other typical characteristics exhibited by most children. By all means get them to tidy up when they have made a mess, but remember there are ways and there are ways ...

You and your partner will need to give each other plenty of support and help during these periods of readjustment. Your partner may want time alone with his or her children, and they may want time alone with your partner just as much. This can be difficult to swallow, because you may feel left out, but it is natural behaviour and you must try to accept it for what it is. There will be times, probably lots of them, when your partner's children are clearly the priority in his or her life. Again, this is a natural response and doesn't mean that you are any less important.

Be considerate of each other's feelings and be tolerant of misunderstandings. Try your hardest not to argue in front of the children, and never make them feel that they are the cause of any argument. Don't forget that your partner is having to come to terms with the changing relationship with his or her own children, too. In time, almost all relationships between children and their parents' new partners settle down, and many turn out to be warm and enduring.

9

building on the relationship

For most live-in relationships to work in the long term, there need to be some basic and consistent foundations. A lot of this book has been devoted to considering how to lay these foundations in practical ways, but now we need also to look at the emotional side of the relationship. It has been said that the best pals and lovers make the best live-in partners. What this means, of course, is that you have to like each other as well as find each other sexually attractive for it to really work. As long as you start off with these prerequisites, you can both do a lot to ensure that the foundations of a good relationship don't crumble as time goes by.

Sharing your life

Although I have advocated the need for each of you to have your own personal space, the whole point of living together is so that you can spend more time in each other's company and do new things together. As well as the trips to the cinema, theatre or restaurants that you may already enjoy on a regular basis, you may discover that you develop an interest in new activities such as going to the gym together or joining a sports club.

More and more, if you consider yourselves as a couple, rather than as two individuals, your friends, relatives and other groups of people will come to regard you in this way, too. Make it clear that this is what you want. If an invitation does not include your partner, be sure to explain to whoever has given the invitation that you have an important other person in your life, and naturally you would like them to come, too, if other guests' spouses are invited. This can apply equally to business as well as social functions. Written acceptance of invitations and thank you notes should indicate the gratitude of both of you – just as it would if you were married.

Occasionally, you may find yourself in a situation where someone is arranging accommodation for you or perhaps just putting you up for the night, but is unaware of your lifestyle. The best course of action is to explain, as soon as is appropriate, that you live – and sleep – together. It will avoid a lot of confusion and embarrassment.

When it comes to giving gifts, those that would normally be given by both a husband and wife together should also be given from both of you. Indeed, in most social situations it is quite acceptable and usual for you to behave in just the same way as a married couple.

With this atmosphere of ready acceptance, it is very easy, over time, to fall into a pattern of behaviour in which the important aspects of the relationship – the very reasons you decided to live together in the first place – get forgotten, or are just pushed conveniently to one side. There are many things you can do towards maintaining values that can help to keep the relationship on a healthy footing.

Respect your partner

First of all, respect your partner's point of view. This doesn't mean you have to agree all the time. It simply means that you give their opinions due consideration. Even if you don't like what's coming, at least hear your partner out when she wants to tell you about her plans to rearrange the whole garden and how you are going to help! Respect also the fact that your partner may require privacy from time to time and may wish to do things that you do not interest you or involve you.

Show true commitment

You don't have to be married to show commitment, despite what some people will tell you. And anyway, as we've already seen, for many people this is not an option. The mere fact that you have set up home together and may have taken on commitments such as a mortgage shows a high level of commitment. Bringing children into the mix raises the level even higher. Showing commitment means being faithful, wanting the same goals, sharing the same values and even discarding past skeletons. It also means always being aware of your own behaviour so that you know how it is impacting on your relationship.

Maintain each other's interest

Try to keep a focus on why the two of you got together in the first place. Almost certainly the main reason was that you were attracted to each other, so try to keep that attraction going. This doesn't mean you have to stay just as you were when you met, of course – as we get older, we all change. Some of us lose our hair and some of us gain weight. But this doesn't mean simply having to give in and let your body go to pieces! Take a pride in your appearance. Try to keep in shape. If we want to, most of us can find the time to exercise more to keep our weight down. We can still eat sensibly and help to avoid piling on the pounds. However old you are, you can still look sexy, distinguished or well turned out if you are prepared to make an effort and dress in a way that pleases both you and your partner.

Keep the old magic going

When it comes to sex, no one expects you to maintain the level of energy you probably had when you first met. But you can always try to be a bit more inventive or adventurous to keep the interest levels high. If you need ideas, there are plenty of books and videos around to show you what to do. Don't be embarrassed about purchasing these; I'm not suggesting you start looking for 'top shelf' material. Many excellent and perfectly respectable guides to better love-making are sold in major bookshops and other outlets and are bought by average, normal couples everywhere.

Of course, the success of your relationship doesn't depend on sex alone. Think back to what else attracted you to your partner – maybe a sense of humour, a determination to get things done, an ability to keep promises no matter what, or a hundred and one other things that make everyone an individual. It's almost certain that your partner was attracted to you for the same sort of reasons and will appreciate being reminded of them now and then. It isn't reasonable to expect you to remember every aspect of your character, but at least try to be the kind of person you were when you first met and do the things that you know please your partner.

Share things

When you live together, you share lots of things as a matter of course – not least your bed and the toothpaste. But there are other ways to share your lives. Share your decisions – those choices you make together are often the best because they mean you both want and get the same thing, which leads to fewer arguments afterwards. Share thoughts with each other, too; in fact, keep communicating as much as you can. Share time together; and try to share interests and common goals. Continue to make your home a shared place. Put pictures of the two of you in the living room and the bedroom. Shop together.

(Just a word of warning, though. It is possible to overdo this sharing stuff – it's called stifling and it's as bad as ignoring your partner and will have the same devastating effect. Moderation, as they say, in all things.)

Stay friends

I know I keep saying this, but it is important to be best friends as well as lovers. If you're still not sure what this means, think of your other good friends; would you ever treat them as badly as you have sometimes treated the person you profess to love the most? I doubt it. Friends support each other and share their problems, they show genuine affection for each other, they boost each other's egos when needed, they are honest with each other, they listen, they cheer each other up, they make time for each other, they put themselves out for each other. Roll just half of that into your relationship with your partner and you're well on the way to long-term success.

Be understanding

It's important to try to understand your partner and look at things from their point of view. It can sometimes be difficult not to nag or want to have things your own way. But remember, it's supposed to be a partnership. I said earlier how important it was to compromise, and it remains important all the way down the line. As time goes on, you'll both change. You will develop new values, new goals and new outlooks. You must learn to respond to each other's new needs and modify your views. You may find yourself wanting your partner to enjoy new things that you have introduced them to. That's fine; it is human nature. But try to avoid turning your partner into someone that they are not. After all, if it is someone else you want, you shouldn't be living with this person.

Show your love

Of course, everything I've just said will help to demonstrate your love for each other, but you can help to keep love healthy in a hundred other little ways. Express your love in words, bring small gifts, make a surprise candle-lit dinner, buy flowers at times other than birthdays or other obvious occasions. Leave messages of love in unexpected places, show your affection by putting your arm around your partner, touch them gently, suggest sex, do something that will delight and excite them – perhaps a surprise weekend away at a romantic seaside hotel or a champagne trip in a hot-air balloon. Get surprise tickets for an important sporting event followed by a slap-up meal. Spending money isn't necessary, however; your partner will appreciate anything if it's fun, original and obviously tailor-made for them. Just giving should please you and will certainly delight the recipient. Consider all this, if you like, as investments in your long-term love account. The more you both put into it, the more you will both get out of it.

Good sex

As I said earlier, keeping love alive doesn't just depend on sex by any means, but it is a vital piece of the jigsaw nevertheless. For most couples, having a good sex life is important and having sex with a committed partner is the best kind of sex. Everyone likes to be told how much they are loved, but most of us prefer action to words! Over time, you will probably discover what turns each of you on the most, and you will no doubt experiment with, and develop, new ways of making love.

You can add all kinds of variety to the experience before you even start making love. What you wear – or don't wear – can make a big impact on your partner, for example. A sexy new hairstyle, new perfume (or aftershave), jewellery and many other things can add that vital sparkle. Whatever you do, don't start taking it – and yourself – too seriously. Laughter is a huge turn-on, in or out of bed.

Don't be surprised if the frequency with which you have sex declines; surveys have shown that it can drop by as much as 25 per cent in four years. And don't expect sex to be an earth-moving experience every time. The desire for sex varies and, like so many things in life, it depends on your mood, whether or not you are tired and many other factors. Sometimes you will want a long, romantic session and at other times you will want a quickie. Again, this is all part of the complex pattern of human nature. By the way, you should remember that sex is good for you! It helps to improve your breathing, cardiovascular system and circulation – it is exercise, after all. It can also release tension and assist the immune system. Having regular sex won't get you fit all by itself, but it is true that if you can stay relatively fit there is a good chance that you will enjoy sex more and maybe more often.

Try to find time for sex, even if you lead busy lives. It's quite natural to feel tired in the evenings during a long working week, and you may have a full social calendar in the evenings at weekends. So, have sex on Saturday morning or in the middle of Sunday afternoon instead. Don't use your lifestyle as a reason not to have sex.

Just a few more thoughts: don't force your attentions on your partner; try to provide sexual satisfaction for your partner during love-making; and don't use withholding sex as a weapon. It's all about consideration, really – but it will pay dividends.

When things go wrong

All couples have disagreements from time to time. Some go further than that and have blazing rows and throw things about. The argument may flare up over something relatively minor or – more seriously – it may be caused by some deep-seated problem that has been simmering for ages. There has been plenty of advice in this book about how to get on in harmony and how to sort out aspects of your lives that can potentially lead to tension. However, each relationship is unique, and only you will know the particular reasons why you are having difficulties.

Small problems, like disagreements about where to place the sofa, can hopefully be sorted out by talking calmly and rationally, or even by indulging in a bit of horse-trading: 'You can have the sofa there, if I can decorate the bathroom the way I want it.' Bigger rows, or ones that seem to loom constantly over all kinds of different issues, may indicate a more profound or even subconscious dissatisfaction with the relationship.

There is no doubt but that cohabitation does bring its own special problems. The trouble may stem from the fact that one of you feels insecure in the relationship. After all, cohabiting does not have the stamp of permanency on it, like marriage. It is important to recognise this, and to avoid making threats such as 'You know I can just leave any time...' that will worsen the situation.

If you think your relationship is beginning to rock dangerously, then maybe you need to do some serious thinking, evaluating and talking. There are plenty of danger signs to look out for:

- You are more relaxed when your partner is not around.
- Your partner's ways and habits are a source of irritation.
- There is little laughter in your home.
- There are constant arguments.
- You are beginning to feel that your partner is no longer the most important person in your world.
- Sexual contact between you seems to be lessening.
- You do not look forward to weekends together.
- You begrudge spending money on the home.
- You do not feel fulfilled in your relationship with your partner.
- You feel stifled by your partner.

You may be experiencing other feelings and emotions, too. We all learn to recognise the signs that tell us all is not as it should be. Or it could be that you sense some of the above in your partner. Either way, if you want the relationship to endure, you must set about finding the root of the problem and then sort it out.

Sometimes, we know what we have done to sour things and, if we are lucky and the wound is not too deep, we can make things better again by simply working hard at mending the relationship. It can be useful to talk to friends and relatives first. They can often supply a more detached view of the situation and may even have observations to offer that had never occurred to you.

Sooner or later, however, you are going to have to talk about the problems with your partner, face to face. In this event, take great care to choose your moment – it should be a time when you know there will not be interruptions and preferably when neither of you is tired or distracted. Try to think through in advance what you want to say and what you want to hear. Although it will be difficult, try very hard not to lose your temper, become over-emotional, make accusations, lie, put all the blame on your partner or belittle them. You must make every effort to remain objective. Be as non-confrontational as possible.

Say 'We' rather than 'I' or 'You' ('I think **we** have a problem', 'Perhaps **we** need to be more honest with each other'.) Try to find out what your partner's views are. Let the discussion take as long as it needs, keep in mind that the reason for the discussion is to solve a problem and talk about how you both think the problem could be solved.

If talking fails to resolve the problem satisfactorily, then you may need to use the services of a relationship counsellor. (Remember, they're not called marriage counsellors any more – they're there for everyone.) Counsellors will usually talk to one or both of you and are trained not only to recognise the problem but also to help you look at and understand the problem, too. They can then offer advice about how you can both work together towards a solution and suggest ways to avoid the problem arising again. You can find counselling services offered in local newspapers, in telephone directories and via institutions such as the Citizens Advice Bureau. There is also counselling advice available on the Internet. It doesn't matter what appears to be the cause of your arguments or disillusionment – sex, money, children, the home or even something you cannot put your finger on – if you think the relationship is worth saving, talk to someone about it. If you don't, things will only get worse and you may end up parting.

10

making a commitment

Some people have a real problem with commitment. Somehow, they say, they feel comfortable to be 'in a relationship' but they don't want to be 'committed' to anyone. It is hard to say why this is so but it's quite likely to be the reason why you are reading this book about living together rather than choosing one about getting married.

Despite this aversion, in reality it is almost impossible to avoid commitment in a relationship. If you are really serious about your partner, then you are almost certainly already committed to them to some extent, even if you don't realise it. As I mentioned in the last chapter, the mere fact that you have decided to live with them indicates a degree of commitment. Your behaviour, if it's loving and considerate, is another sign of your commitment. And, of course, it doesn't have to go any further than that, if you don't want it to. There's no reason why you can't just move in together and then keep the relationship alive just as it is, for ever, is there? Well, actually, I think there is.

It is a statistical fact that those who choose to make the commitment of marriage are more likely to stay together than those who choose merely to live together. So it would appear that there is something in that ceremony, those vows made in public, that strengthens the ties between two people. And if that's the case, it probably makes sense for couples who want to forge a lasting relationship, albeit without getting married, to consider undertaking something similar in order to cement the bonds of their liaison.

For whatever reason, more and more couples living together nowadays decide that they want to make some sort of public pledge to each other. This is an excellent idea, in my opinion. It provides an ideal opportunity for you to show your family and friends that you are serious about this relationship – that it is more to you than just a casual fling. That in itself will probably please your parents and other older relatives but what is more important is that it shows that you are willing to demonstrate what you really feel, in front of people who matter to you. Making a promise in private is one thing. Making a public declaration is quite another, and it will carry even more weight if you know that the people witnessing it are closely acquainted with you and will remind you of it.

On a more intimate level, it will, almost certainly, make you and your partner think even harder about your reasons for choosing each other and deciding to live together. In the future, your declaration to each other in public will become a focal point in your relationship. It will give you concrete reasons for staying together and it will provide you with something to help you get over the problems that, inevitably, will occur.

Marking the occasion

There is no doubt that making a public commitment to your partner is a serious business. But there is a fun side too, which involves how and where you are going to mark the occasion and celebrate it. This is better known as having a party, and here the possibilities and permutations are endless. The event can be as large or as small, as simple or as elaborate as you want. You could have a small family dinner party or a big bash with a disco for all your relatives and everyone you know, a barbecue in the garden or a fancy outing to the top of the Eiffel Tower... The choice really is entirely up to you. It has to be said that it all sounds rather like a wedding reception – and certainly you'll find that wedding books and magazines are an excellent source of ideas for how to celebrate. But in many ways there is far more scope for you and your partner to make it unique to you.

That word 'unique' is important. The key to getting the occasion right is making sure that it feels special and comfortable for you both. Unlike a wedding, when the whole organisation is often hijacked by the mother of the bride, this day is strictly for you and your partner, so you can organise it and do it just as you like. You can plan every detail and lay down formal arrangements or you can make it entirely informal and open-ended. You don't even have to tell your guests the purpose of the party if you don't want to – just invite everyone round and then spring it on them on the day. A word of warning, however: you may want it to be a casual event, and you may feel the less it is like a conventional marriage ceremony, the better. But your guests may not be entirely happy with this unstructured approach. A surprising number of people prefer to have an established etiquette to follow – what to wear, whether they should bring a present and so on. Be unconventional, if that's what you want, but it's probably best if you tell everyone what you have in mind.

Making the arrangements

One of the reasons you may have decided simply to live together is that you didn't want all the hassle of going through a wedding ceremony, organising the reception and coping with everything that involves. If that's so, you may find the next few paragraphs rather trying because no matter how relaxed and informal you may want it to be, every party requires some planning. You and your partner will have to put your heads together and make a few decisions. For a start, you must agree on how much you want to spend: this will depend on the sort of occasion you want, and particularly on the level of formality. You'll need to choose and possibly book the location, decide whether you are going to send out invitations, think about who is going to provide the food and drink, and so on. It will probably help to remind yourselves that you can do everything exactly as you want – there is no one to please but each other.

You will also have to draw up a guest list. This is a potential minefield – if you restrict it to very close family members you risk offending someone, and if you issue an open invitation to everyone you know you may find that the whole purpose of the day gets lost. You probably hoped you'd avoided all this kind of thing by not getting married in the first place. But there is a way round it and, once again, the trick is to decide what sort of occasion you want, and work from there. Keep reminding yourself why you are organising the event in the first place: decide which people are important to **you**, and exactly who you want to be present on this special day. These are the only people you need to invite – whether you want six or 60, that's entirely up to you.

You and your partner must also decide if you are going to actually stand up and speak. Since the whole idea is that you are going to mark the occasion by making a public statement of your commitment to each other, one or both of you will almost certainly have to say something. You may even want to make vows. Again, don't be put off by this suggestion because you don't want it to be like a wedding or any kind of religious occasion. Making vows doesn't have to be either of these – lots of people make vows in secular ceremonies, expressing their intentions and feelings towards to each other, so you can take ideas from them.

Whatever you are going to say, plan it in advance, preferably with your partner. You can use whatever words you think are appropriate but don't make it too long. A few words spoken from the heart are much better than a long speech that you struggle to remember or, worse still, have to read from a piece of paper. It is a good idea to make clear to your guests what is going to happen and ask them to remain quiet while you go through what you want to say – if you are taking this seriously, so should they.

Looking back – and forward

Once it's all over, you will realise that you have something very precious to look back on. In addition, now that you have established this day as a special occasion, it will provide you with a reason celebrate its anniversary every year. Don't be put off by the word 'anniversary' because you're anti-weddings. After all, it will be a good excuse for a party every time it comes round. But, more seriously, you and your partner can use the occasion to remind each other about your good times and to resolve any issues outstanding over the bad times. It will provide you each year with a time to think about why you are together and what is special about your relationship – and why you want to make it last.

11

where do we go from here?

If you intend to stay with your partner for life, there will almost certainly come a point in your relationship when you have to make a positive decision about your future together. The choice is simple: you either carry on indefinitely as you are – a perfectly valid option – or you get married.

So, despite the fact that this is a book about cohabiting, I think it's appropriate here to give some space to discussing the merits and pitfalls of matrimony.

To marry or not to marry

There are many similarities between living together and marriage, but there are also many differences. Some, as we have seen, are legal and financial differences, and others relate to the different perceptions and values placed on these two states by society. But there is much more. Most of the important differences are the ones that you must want to embrace and experience as a couple. Living together and marriage call for different mind-sets. If you think you want to move from cohabiting to marriage, you should not only be ready and eager to accept these mind-set changes, you should already be feeling some of them and sensing that for you, marriage is the only way forward. Marriage, it must be said, involves extra responsibilities, commitments, financial intertwining, expectations and general 'relationship upgrading', for want of a better phrase. If you think you want to get married, you must be sure that you want these too.

Added to that, for a marriage to work, you have **both** got to want to be married. Neither of you should feel that one is coercing the other into marriage.

Even more importantly, you should not just drift into marriage because you hope it will rejuvenate a flagging live-in relationship. It won't. It will just add to the problems. Take a good look at yourself if you have any doubts about this. Do you value a fairly high degree of independence (both financially and personally)? Do you prefer to keep your partner's family at arm's length? Is your social and financial background very different from your partner's? Does living together suit you just fine? If the answer to any of these is 'Yes', then there's a good chance that marriage is not going to be right for you.

Saying 'Yes'

Before making this next big step, it does no harm to talk things through with others who have chosen this path. If you are lucky, you may know married friends who started by living together. If not, at least talk to as many married couples as you feel necessary to get a view on this new (for you) kind of relationship. Ask them about how the everyday things in their life work as a married couple, and compare the answers with your situation now. (Who does the shopping? Who makes the bed? Does she mind him going out to the pub? What does he do when she wants to have a girlfriend round for a girly night in?) How do you feel about the differences? If you are having trouble with your decision, you can go for premarital counselling, just like the counselling you get to help resolve relationship difficulties. If it becomes clear from this that your relationship will suffer if you get married, as is sometimes the case, it may prevent you from making a big mistake.

If you and your partner are both firmly set on the idea of marriage, then go for it! A good marriage should enhance all the best things about your cohabiting relationship as well as introduce you to a whole new set of experiences. You should enjoy a relationship that increases your contentment, helps you get closer to your goals in life, fulfils you emotionally and physically and opens new doors for you. Many couples arrange for the occasion of their marriage to coincide with some other important event in their lives – moving house, changing jobs, announcing a pregnancy or taking a special holiday, for example. This can help to make the timing of the marriage even more momentous and meaningful; the beginning of a new life chapter.

It won't all be a bed of roses unless you are still prepared to work at it, however. It is unlikely that your new spouse will be any better disposed towards your bad habits than when they were your live-in lover, so don't go thinking you can just do as you please now you are married. All those words like respect, commitment and trust mean just as much now as they did before you were married. Because many of the expectations in marriage are different from those in cohabitation, it can be difficult to adjust to the changes initially. Inevitably, the relationship you have with each other will now alter.

Marriage, just like cohabitation, is a partnership, but as you will quickly find, it is a different sort of partnership. You may find one or other of you taking the lead in certain decision-making processes that you used to do together, for example. Your partner may expect to have more say over certain aspects of your life. The way your finances work may change. You will certainly need to consider your spouse first and foremost. But then these are some of the reasons why you wanted to get married, aren't they?

And if it's a 'No'

Inevitably, some live-in relationships are doomed to fail. You have tried your best, you have talked it through, but the differences seem irreconcilable. All you can do now is resign yourself to the situation and try to make the break-up as painless as possible for both of you. It's time to close this chapter in your life. Although there is bound to be sadness and a feeling of loss and even failure, in time these feelings should subside, and you may come to realise that an unhappy or pointless relationship is not in your interests any more than your partner's.

Disentangling the wreckage

Breaking up is not easy. It requires time and attention and you would probably prefer to ignore anything and everything to do with your partner. Don't do this. Apart from the emotional traumas and the other people to consider, such as children, there may also be financial and legal issues to sort out, as well as the problem of deciding how to divide up any shared assets. Even if you rent a property, you cannot just walk out when it suits you – or at least you shouldn't. Your lease is probably subject to a contract, which stipulates that you must pay the rent for a given period of time. Although you may be able to vacate the property early, the chances are you will still have to pay for the full term of the lease. It is possible that one or other of you wants to stay in the property, in which case you may have to renegotiate the tenancy with the landlord. If the rent has been paid in advance, the person staying in the property will need to reimburse the person moving out.

If you have bought your own home as a couple, you will need to decide whether you will sell it and share the proceeds, or whether one of you will remain in the property and give the other a cash sum to buy out their share. Then there are all the things you bought jointly to sort out. If you made a record of all of these things as I suggested earlier, then this part of the proceedings should be fairly straightforward and relatively painless.

The whole thing will be much less painful if you get yourselves organised to make decisions – together. It will help if you can decide when the split is actually going to take place. Factors that affect this will include lease renewal dates, the need to find alternative accommodation, the sale of a jointly owned property, schooling arrangements for children and so on. It may be best to draw up some form of documentation setting out the timing of events. If your partner is stonewalling, you can do this on your own – then give them a copy.

If you have entered into any financial or legal arrangements of which your partner was a beneficiary – for example, a will or insurance policies – it will be necessary to inform the relevant bodies or companies so that you can make any necessary amendments. Don't forget about credit agreements and any other similar commitments that may need reviewing in the light of your impending break-up. For example, if you are paying for the washing machine by instalments, are you going to take it with you if you move out?

Tell your friends and family about your plans. Don't put this off – you will have to do it sooner or later and you may want to call on them for both moral support and for help when it comes to actually moving out. Perhaps your family may even be able to provide short-term financial assistance if required. Friends and family can also be very welcome at a time when you may be feeling very vulnerable and under siege. They can often look at things from a slightly different perspective and may be able to give you useful advice or suggest courses of action you had not considered.

If you are both moving out of a property, you should each pack your own belongings, making sure that everything is clearly marked – especially things placed in sealed boxes – so that there is no confusion as to the ownership of items. On the actual day you move out, try to remain amicable if your ex-partner is still around. Call on that friend or family member if you need extra support. If the place needs cleaning up, insist that your ex-partner helps. By the same token, of course, if you're moving out and your partner isn't, you shouldn't leave the place like a pigsty.

Helping children cope

Break-ups are particularly difficult for children. Their feelings must also be considered if you and your partner are breaking up. The law usually provides for continuing financial support from both biological parents and for residence with the natural mother (see Chapter 8). However, there is much you can both do to ease their pain in the event of a break-up by trying to avoid having arguments in their presence and by generally maintaining a positive outlook for them. Many of the strategies adopted to help children to understand and cope when their married parents part are equally relevant in this situation, of course (see page 85).

It is also worth bearing in mind that it may still be better for them in the long term to be in a new environment that is free from the bickering and the generally sullied atmosphere that prevails in a relationship that is breaking down.

Life goes on

When the final break has happened, and you and your one-time partner no longer live under the same roof, the healing process can begin. Don't look on this as failure on your part. It has happened to millions of people everywhere, and it will happen to millions more.

Most people go through stages of unhappiness, recrimination, guilt and sorrow after finishing a close relationship, but the best way to get over these feelings quickly is to start your life afresh. See your friends, go out whenever you are invited, do some of the things you always wanted to do, buy some new clothes or treat yourself to a makeover, tell yourself that your ex-partner made mistakes as well as you.

Take the time to analyse the events of the past, but don't dwell on them for too long. Instead, come to terms with and reconcile yourself to the fact that the relationship is over. Keep reminding yourself that finding the right person takes, amongst other things, a great deal of luck. So you just haven't been lucky up until now – but you might be next time.

further information

There are many books and other publications available that can provide advice on almost all aspects of a living-together relationship. There are also advice centres and other professional bodies ready to help. Many of these have their own websites where services on offer can be located, or where information and advice is available on screen. Some of the most useful sources are listed below and on page 108.

Books

Gray, J, *Men Are From Mars, Women Are from Venus*, Thorsons, 1993
Hunt, A E, *Loving Someone Else's Child*, iUniverse, 2000
Kitchen, G, *Check Your Tax and Money Facts*, Foulsham, 2002
Mack, L, *Setting Up Home*, Carlton Books, 2000
Melledy, P, *Facing Love Addiction*, Harper San Francisco, 1992
Quilliam, S, *Staying Together*, Vermilion, 2001
Rosen, R, *The Complete Idiot's Guide to Living Together*, Alpha Books, 2001
Stanway, A, *The Lovers' Guide*, Pan MacMillan, 1992
Stoddart, A, *Living Beautifully Together*, Avon Books, 1991
Wilson, H, *Money Matters*, Pan, 1981

Websites

Relationship issues

www.candis.co.uk – parenting and relationships

www.oneplusone.org.uk – marriage and relationships

www.opfs.org – One Parent Families in Scotland site – and www.spig.clara.net – Shared Parenting Information Group site – information and advice on issues relating to children

Legal and financial matters

www.adviceguide.org.uk – Citizens Advice Bureau* site, offering factual information and advice on a wide range of issues

www.law4today.com – legal advice and tips, including the likely cost of various legal transactions

www.lawsociety.org.uk and www.lawscot.org.uk – sites for the Law Society, offering information on all aspects of lawyers and the law, including a list of solicitors* belonging to the Society's Children Panel

www.sfla.co.uk – Solicitors Family Law Association site

www.inlandrevenue.gov.uk – Inland Revenue* site, full of information and guidance on tax matters

www.find.co.uk – information directory, plus guidance on investments, insurance, savings, loans and financial advice

www.dss.gov.uk – Benefits Agency* (Department of Social Security) site with information on benefits and how to apply for them

If you do not have access to the Internet, those organisations marked * may be found in your local telephone directory or Yellow Pages.

index